KILLED BY FRAGRANCE

How Synthetic Scents Make Us Sick

Dr. Joseph Jacobs, DPT, ACN

First Edition, February 2026
Published by ASTR Institute
614 E HWY 50 #169, Clermont, FL 34711

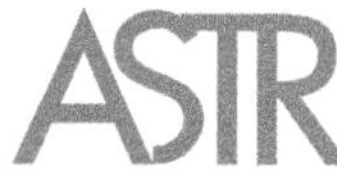

ASTRinstitute.com

Disclaimer

This book, authored by Dr. Joseph Jacobs and published by the ASTR Institute, is intended for informational purposes only and presents medical research findings. It is not a substitute for professional medical advice, diagnosis, or treatment. Dr. Joseph Jacobs, the ASTR Institute, and its affiliates do not endorse or assume responsibility for any specific medical treatments or procedures discussed in this book. We strongly advise readers to consult with their healthcare providers regarding the applicability of any aspects of the content to their own health and well-being.

The statements contained herein have not been evaluated by the Food and Drug Administration. The products mentioned are not designed to diagnose, cure, treat, or prevent any disease. Individual results may vary, and we cannot guarantee that you will achieve the same outcomes as those detailed in our case studies, testimonials, and treatment videos. Success varies per individual, and one person's results do not guarantee similar outcomes for another.
If you have medical concerns, consult with your healthcare provider, physician, or another qualified medical professional. Dr. Joseph Jacobs, the ASTR Institute, and their associated organizations and individuals disclaim any liability for actions, services, or products acquired through this book, our videos, website, or any of our media channels.

Table of Contents

Online Resources

How to Access Online Resources

Throughout this book, you'll find barcodes that link to additional online resources. Here's how to use them:

1. Open the camera app on your smartphone.
2. Point the camera at the barcode.
3. A notification will appear with a link. Tap the notification to open the link in your browser.

My Fragrance Story

My Fragrance Story: From Survival to Purpose

After my second cancer treatment, I began to notice something unsettling. Everyday fragrances that I had once barely registered suddenly felt overwhelming. At first, the change was subtle. Then it intensified. Environments saturated with synthetic fragrances became physiologically intolerable. Certain facilities triggered immediate and severe reactions. What began as discomfort escalated into debilitating migraines, panic-like episodes, and pronounced respiratory and allergic symptoms. I experienced intense nasal congestion, shortness of breath, a burning sore throat, coughing, sneezing, and watery, painful eyes. These reactions were not fleeting or mild. They were reproducible, disruptive, and resolved only after removal from exposure.

As the symptoms worsened, I became determined to understand what was happening. Through careful observation, I identified consistent patterns associated with fragranced environments. That discovery led to a deeper question: Was I alone in this experience?

I searched for books addressing fragrance sensitivity and chemical exposure, hoping to find validation or guidance. I found nothing. When I turned to the scientific literature, however, the data were striking.

Multiple population studies report that **approximately 20 to 34 percent of adults experience adverse health effects** from fragranced products. Reported symptoms include headaches, migraines, asthma exacerbations, respiratory distress, neurological complaints, skin irritation, and allergic reactions. This pattern is not rare. It is widespread, underrecognized, and frequently minimized. Seeing these numbers stopped me in my tracks. When nearly one third of adults report health effects from fragranced products, the issue can no longer be dismissed as isolated sensitivity. It represents a significant public health concern. That realization compelled me to write this book.

Killed by Fragrance exists to examine the evidence, validate lived experiences, and bring visibility to a largely unaddressed health issue. Throughout this book, I have intentionally included peer-reviewed studies and referenced data in every section. Fragrance-related illness is often minimized because it is misunderstood. Evidence provides clarity. Science gives structure to lived experience. Data demand accountability.

My hope is that this book equips readers with knowledge and restores confidence in their own physiological responses. Regulatory agencies, healthcare systems, and workplaces have an opportunity to implement protective policies grounded in evidence. Awareness is the first step. Action must follow.

If you recognize yourself in these pages, consider using this book as a professional resource. Share it with legislators. Provide it to healthcare administrators. Present it to workplace leadership and human resources departments. It was written and extensively researched to function in these settings.

When **nearly one third of adults report adverse effects**, the issue warrants serious consideration. It should not be dismissed. It should be examined, addressed, and responsibly regulated.

Truth has power. It is time for that truth to inform meaningful change.

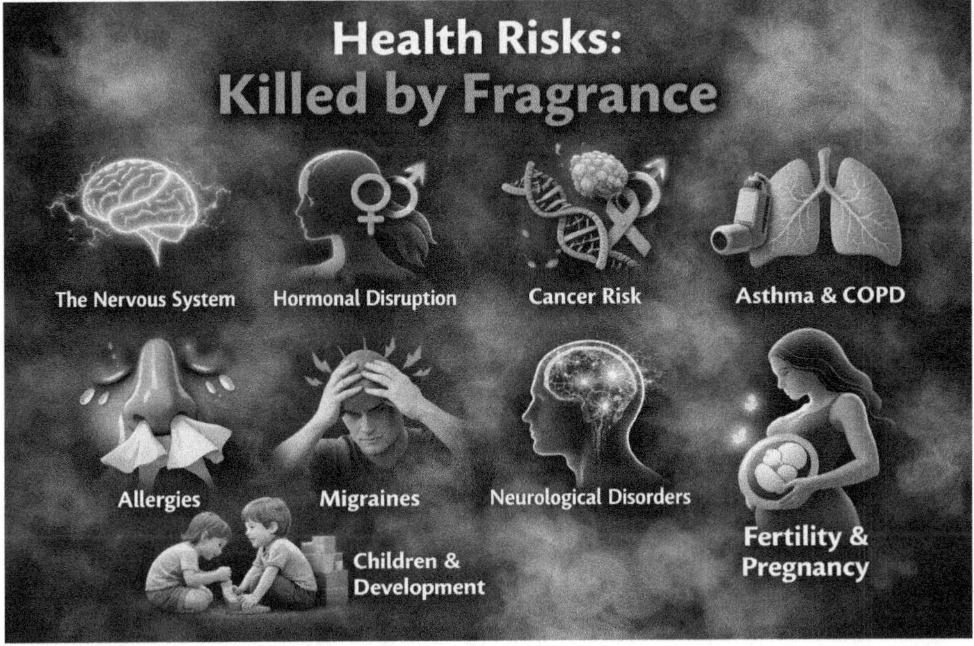
Health Risks:
Killed by Fragrance
The Nervous System
Hormonal Disruption
Cancer Risk
Asthma & COPD
Allergies
Migraines
Neurological Disorders
Children &
Development
Fertility &
Pregnancy

When Fragrance Is Not Benign: Documented Cases of Severe Harm

Fragranced products are widely perceived as harmless consumer goods. They are marketed as symbols of cleanliness, comfort, and personal identity. However, clinical and public health literature tells a very different story. While not every exposure results in harm, there are documented cases in which fragranced products have caused severe medical emergencies, permanent disability, and even death. These cases reveal a critical truth: fragrance exposure is not biologically neutral, and for some individuals, it is profoundly dangerous. This chapter examines real, published cases that demonstrate how fragranced products can trigger life-threatening reactions through toxic, immunologic, neurologic, and cardiopulmonary pathways.

Acute Anaphylaxis and Respiratory Failure

One of the clearest demonstrations of fragrance-related medical danger is acute anaphylaxis. In a peer-reviewed case report, a healthcare worker experienced a sudden anaphylactic reaction after being sprayed in the face with perfume at work. The exposure triggered severe bronchospasm, airway compromise, and prolonged respiratory symptoms requiring aggressive medical treatment (Lessenger, 2001). Importantly, this individual did not have a known prior allergy to perfume. The reaction occurred through inhalation and mucosal exposure alone, underscoring that fragrance chemicals can act as potent triggers capable of overwhelming immune and respiratory defenses in susceptible individuals. Additional cases reinforce this pathway, including reports of anaphylactoid reactions, severe respiratory distress, and rare systemic effects like urticaria from fragrance inhalation, even in individuals without prior sensitization (Elberling et al., 2005; Novak-Bilić et al., 2018).

Cardiac Arrhythmia Following Aerosol Exposure

Fragrance-related harm is not limited to allergic pathways. In a striking case published in The Journal of Electrocardiology, a young woman collapsed after an air freshener was sprayed directly into her nostrils. She was found to be in ventricular fibrillation, a life-threatening cardiac arrhythmia requiring immediate defibrillation to prevent death (Senthilkumaran et al., 2012). Chemical analysis identified hydrocarbon propellants, including isobutane, as the likely contributors. This case illustrates that inhaled fragrance products, particularly aerosols, can disrupt cardiac electrical activity through toxic and autonomic mechanisms. The authors aptly titled their report "Death Just a Breath Away," reflecting the severity and immediacy of the risk.

Fatal Poisoning From Household Air Fresheners

Fragranced products also pose lethal risks through ingestion, whether accidental or intentional. A forensic autopsy report described the death of an elderly man following ingestion of a repellent air freshener. Toxicologic findings and tissue damage confirmed fatal poisoning attributable to the product's chemical constituents (Hitosugi et al., 2015). While ingestion is often dismissed as misuse, these products are sold without adequate warnings and are frequently present in homes with children, cognitively impaired adults, and elderly individuals. Their chemical composition is far from benign.

Fatal Infections Linked to Aromatherapy Products

In 2021, a Centers for Disease Control and Prevention investigation identified a rare and deadly bacterial infection linked to a commercially sold aromatherapy room spray. The product, sold nationwide, was contaminated with Burkholderia pseudomallei, a pathogen capable of causing melioidosis, a frequently fatal disease. Four confirmed infections occurred in the United States, resulting in two deaths (Centers for Disease Control and Prevention, 2021). This case is particularly alarming because it involved a product marketed as "natural," "essential oil–based," and wellness-oriented. The outbreak led to a nationwide recall by the U.S. Consumer Product Safety Commission, confirming that fragranced products can pose risks far beyond chemical toxicity alone. Follow-up reports confirmed the spray's role in additional fatalities, including a child, and even the death of a pet exposed in the home (CDC, 2022).

Occupational Asthma and Repeated Emergency Care

Fragrance exposure is a well-documented trigger of occupational asthma. Surveillance data from California identified hundreds of confirmed work-related asthma cases associated with fragranced products, including perfumes, colognes, and air fresheners. Many of these cases involved new-onset asthma, not merely exacerbation of preexisting disease (Weinberg et al., 2017). From 1993–2012, California surveillance documented 270 work-related asthma cases linked to fragrances, representing 3.8% of all confirmed cases, often from coworker or environmental exposures (California Department of Public Health, 2020). In documented examples, workers developed severe asthma attacks immediately following fragrance exposure at work, requiring emergency department visits and systemic steroid treatment. In some cases, repeated exposures led to job loss because symptoms became unmanageable in fragranced environments (California Department of Public Health, 2017). Recent reviews highlight occupational risks in beauty salons, spas, and manufacturing, where prolonged inhalation of concentrated mixtures contributes to chronic respiratory conditions (Manful et al., 2024). These cases demonstrate that fragrance-related illness is not rare, psychological, or subjective. It is diagnosable, reportable, and preventable.

What These Cases Reveal

Taken together, these cases demonstrate several critical points: First, fragranced products can cause harm through multiple biological mechanisms, including immune activation, neurogenic inflammation, toxic inhalation, and cardiac instability. Second, serious outcomes can occur in both previously healthy individuals and those with underlying vulnerability. **Prior tolerance does not guarantee future safety**. Third, the risks are not confined to extreme misuse. Many exposures occurred in ordinary environments such as workplaces, homes, and retail settings. Finally, these harms are underrecognized because fragrance ingredients are poorly disclosed, regulatory oversight is limited, and symptoms are often dismissed or misattributed.

Research and Studies: The Scientific Evidence on Synthetic Fragrance

Synthetic fragrance exposure represents a significant and underrecognized public health issue. Fragranced consumer products are used daily across personal care, cleaning, healthcare, occupational, and public environments. Despite their widespread use, the chemical constituents of synthetic fragrances are largely undisclosed, insufficiently tested as mixtures, and associated with a growing body of evidence documenting adverse health effects across multiple organ systems.

The term fragrance or perfume does not denote a single compound. It is a legally protected trade secret that can contain dozens to hundreds of individual chemicals, including volatile organic compounds, solvents, preservatives, fixatives, and known endocrine active substances (Steinemann, 2016). Manufacturers are not required to disclose these components on product labels, even when products are marketed as natural, unscented, or green. This limits informed consumer choice and complicates exposure assessment.

Population-Level Evidence

Epidemiological studies consistently demonstrate that a substantial proportion of the population reports adverse health effects associated with fragranced product exposure. In nationally representative surveys conducted in the United States, Australia, the United Kingdom, and Sweden, **approximately one third of adults reported health problems attributed to fragranced products**. Reported symptoms included headaches, migraines, respiratory distress, asthma attacks, skin reactions, neurological symptoms, and cognitive impairment (Steinemann et al., 2016; Steinemann, 2018). These effects were reported by individuals with and without preexisting medical conditions. Among respondents with asthma, adverse reactions were significantly more prevalent. In one study, more than **sixty percent of asthmatics reported respiratory symptoms triggered by fragranced products,** compared with fewer than twenty five percent of nonasthmatics (Steinemann et al., 2019). These findings have been replicated across multiple countries, suggesting that fragrance sensitivity reflects a widespread exposure-related phenomenon rather than isolated intolerance. Recent **international surveys** and reviews (2020–2025) confirm **20–35% of adults experience fragrance-related health effects**, often leading to social isolation, restricted access to public spaces, lost workdays, or job loss, with respiratory problems predominant (Steinemann, 2021; Forced isolation by invisible barriers, 2025; Martins et al., 2023).

Chemical Emissions and Indoor Air Quality

Analytical chemistry studies using gas chromatography mass spectrometry have identified more than one hundred distinct volatile organic compounds emitted from common fragranced consumer products. These include air fresheners, laundry detergents, dryer sheets, and personal care items (Steinemann, 2011).

Many of these compounds are classified as hazardous air pollutants under United States federal law, including acetaldehyde, formaldehyde, benzene derivatives, and terpenes. Indoor chemistry further amplifies risk. Terpenes such as limonene and alpha pinene, commonly used for fragrance, react with indoor ozone to form secondary pollutants. These include formaldehyde and ultrafine particulate matter. These secondary compounds are associated with airway irritation, oxidative stress, and inflammatory responses (Weschler & Shields, 1997; Nazaroff & Weschler, 2004). Emerging research (2024–2025) shows fragranced products actively alter indoor air chemistry, forming nanoparticles at high concentrations when terpenes react with ozone, penetrating deep into the respiratory system and posing risks to lung health, with particle concentrations rivaling those from combustion sources like gas stoves or diesel engines (Jung et al., 2025; Purdue University study, 2025; Katam et al., 2025). Scented wax melts, with higher fragrance oil concentrations, produce significantly more nanoparticles than candles (ACS ES&T Letters, 2025).

Respiratory Effects

The respiratory system is among the most consistently affected targets of synthetic fragrance exposure. Controlled exposure studies and clinical observations demonstrate that inhalation of fragranced volatile organic compounds can provoke bronchoconstriction, mucosal irritation, and exacerbation of asthma and chronic obstructive pulmonary disease (Caress & Steinemann, 2009). Even low-level exposures have been associated with measurable declines in pulmonary function and increased symptom burden in susceptible individuals (Anderson & Anderson, 1998). Healthcare environments are of particular concern. Studies report that fragranced products used in hospitals and clinics can trigger respiratory symptoms in patients and staff. This undermines patient safety and occupational health (Ziem & McTamney, 1997). Recent assessments link fragrance emissions to elevated PM2.5, formaldehyde, and TVOC levels indoors, with hazard quotients indicating carcinogenic and non-carcinogenic risks from chronic inhalation, including sinus inflammation and breathing difficulties (Katam et al., 2025; Ohio State Health & Discovery, 2023; Martins et al., 2023).

Neurological and Cognitive Effects

Neurological symptoms including headaches, migraines, dizziness, nausea, anxiety, and cognitive fog are among the most frequently reported outcomes of fragrance exposure. Experimental and clinical research suggests that fragrance chemicals activate the trigeminal nerve and limbic system. These regions are involved in pain perception, autonomic regulation, and emotional processing (Doty et al., 2004). Fragrance-induced migraines are well documented in headache literature, with scent exposure recognized as a common and potent trigger. Neurogenic inflammation and sensory hypersensitization provide biologically plausible mechanisms for these effects (Kelman, 2007). Reviews highlight neurotoxicity from phthalates, synthetic musks, and sensitizers, contributing to headaches, depression, cognitive issues, and potential long-term brain impacts (Kovalchuk et al., 2018; Martins et al., 2023; Li et al., 2024).

Endocrine and Hormonal Disruption

A substantial body of research identifies fragrance ingredients as endocrine disrupting chemicals. Phthalates, widely used as fragrance fixatives, exhibit estrogenic and antiandrogenic activity. They have been associated with altered thyroid function, impaired fertility, insulin resistance, developmental abnormalities, and reproductive toxicity in epidemiological and experimental studies (Meeker et al., 2009; Gore et al., 2015). Synthetic musks represent another class of fragrance compounds of concern. These chemicals are lipophilic and bioaccumulative. They have been detected in human adipose tissue, breast milk, and umbilical cord blood. These findings raise concerns regarding chronic exposure, hormonal interference, and developmental vulnerability (Reiner et al., 2007). Recent analyses confirm phthalates, parabens, and synthetic musks in fragranced products disrupt estrogen, androgen, and thyroid pathways, linking to reproductive issues, cancer risks, metabolic disorders, insulin resistance, and miscarriage odds in human studies (Frontiers in Toxicology, 2025; MDPI Endocrines, 2024; Breast Cancer Prevention Partners, 2025; Burkart, 2025).

Immune, Dermatologic, and Sensitization Effects

Fragrance chemicals are among the most common causes of allergic contact dermatitis worldwide. Patch testing studies consistently identify fragrance mixtures as leading sensitizers, with prevalence increasing over time (Basketter et al., 2019). Beyond classic allergic mechanisms, fragrance exposure has been associated with non-IgE mediated immune activation. This is consistent with irritant-induced inflammation and chemical sensitivity syndromes. Fragrance allergens affect 2–11% of the population, with oxidized forms of limonene and linalool prominent (de Groot, 2021). Recent data (2019–2025) show fragrances remain highly prevalent allergens in cosmetics, with positivity rates of 5–25% in patch-tested patients and up to 12.8% for fragrance mix I in North American studies; "natural" products often contain multiple allergens (NACDG, 2019–2020; What is New in Contact Allergy To Cosmetics, 2025; JAMA Dermatology, 2022).

Cancer and Long-Term Toxicity

Certain fragrance constituents and secondary reaction products exhibit mutagenic or carcinogenic properties in laboratory studies. Formaldehyde releasers, benzene derivatives, and polycyclic musks have been classified or evaluated as carcinogenic or potentially carcinogenic by international agencies (International Agency for Research on Cancer, 2012). While establishing direct causality in human populations is complex, chronic low-dose exposure and bioaccumulation raise legitimate concerns. This is especially relevant given the absence of long-term safety testing for fragrance mixtures (Kortenkamp & Faust, 2018). Recent product testing and risk assessments flag high concerns for cancer, genetic mutations, and chronic toxicity from undisclosed fragrance chemicals, with 48 ingredients showing established high hazards including mammary carcinogens (Breast Cancer Prevention Partners, 2025).

Converging Evidence

Across epidemiological surveys, chemical analyses, toxicological experiments, clinical case reports, and occupational studies, a consistent pattern emerges. Synthetic fragrance exposure is associated with multisystem health effects involving the respiratory, neurological, endocrine, immune, and dermatologic systems. These findings are biologically supported, reproducible, and increasingly documented in peer-reviewed literature. The scientific question is no longer whether synthetic fragrance exposure can cause harm. The evidence demonstrates that it can and does. The more pressing issue is why such exposures remain normalized, underregulated, and insufficiently disclosed in modern environments.

The scientific literature consistently demonstrates that synthetic fragrance exposure is associated with multisystem health effects. Epidemiological, toxicological, and clinical evidence converge to show that fragrance-related illness is widespread, biologically supported, and underrecognized. The question is no longer whether harm exists, but why these exposures remain normalized and insufficiently regulated.

What Fragrance Is

Fragrance is one of the most poorly understood and least transparent components of modern consumer products. While commonly perceived as a benign additive meant to improve smell, fragrance is in fact a complex chemical system intentionally designed to disperse into air, adhere to surfaces, and interact with the human body. Understanding what fragrance actually is is essential to understanding its health effects.

The Meaning of the Term Fragrance

In consumer product labeling, the terms fragrance and perfume do not represent a single substance. They refer to proprietary chemical mixtures that may contain dozens to hundreds of individual compounds. These mixtures are protected under trade secret laws, allowing manufacturers to withhold full ingredient disclosure from product labels and safety documentation (Steinemann, 2016). **Analytical studies have demonstrated that fragranced products often emit chemicals not listed on labels, including volatile organic compounds (VOCs) classified as hazardous under federal law** (Steinemann, 2011; Steinemann, 2015). This lack of transparency limits consumer choice, complicates clinical evaluation, and obscures exposure assessment in epidemiological research. Recent regulatory developments, such as the EU's 2023 amendment expanding mandatory disclosure of fragrance allergens from 26 to over 80 compounds (effective 2026 for new products), aim to address this, though full ingredient lists remain limited in many regions (Regulation (EU) 2023/1545; IFRA, 2025).

Where Fragrance Is Hiding: Everyday Products That Contain Scented Chemical Mixtures

- Perfume and cologne
- Body sprays and deodorant
- Soap and body wash
- Shampoo and conditioner
- Hair styling products
- Lotions and moisturizers
- Sunscreen
- Shaving products
- Makeup and cosmetics

- Baby care products
- Feminine hygiene products
- Laundry detergent and fabric softeners
- Household cleaning products
- Air fresheners and scented candles
- Essential oil and diffuser blends
- Hotel and spa toiletries
- Commercial and institutional cleaning agents
- Automotive interior products and air fresheners
- Scented paper goods and trash bags
- Cat litter
- Mattress and fabric sprays
- New clothing finishing treatments
- Hand sanitizers and antibacterial soaps
- Disinfectant wipes and sprays
- Certain topical medications and medical products

Composition of Fragrance Mixtures

Fragrance formulations typically include solvents, stabilizers, preservatives, fixatives, and volatile scent compounds. These chemicals are selected not only for their odor but also for their ability to evaporate efficiently, persist over time, and remain stable across diverse product applications. A single fragrance formulation may be used across perfumes, lotions, detergents, cleaning products, and air fresheners, increasing cumulative exposure from multiple sources. Studies using gas chromatography mass spectrometry have identified more than one hundred distinct volatile organic compounds emitted from fragranced consumer products, many of which are not disclosed on product labels (Steinemann, 2011; Steinemann, 2015). These include terpenes, aldehydes, and petroleum-derived solvents. Recent analyses confirm that even "green" or "natural" labeled products emit similar VOC profiles, including hazardous air pollutants (Steinemann, 2015).

Natural and Synthetic Fragrance

Fragrance ingredients may be derived from natural sources, synthetic sources, or a combination of both. Natural fragrance compounds are often extracted from plants through distillation or solvent extraction. However, natural origin does not equate to safety. Many naturally derived fragrance compounds, such as limonene and linalool in essential oils, are potent sensitizers or irritants, particularly when concentrated or oxidized (de Groot, 2021). Recent narrative reviews highlight that **natural fragrances can trigger allergic contact dermatitis and respiratory issues comparable to synthetics** (Martins et al., 2023; Ahmed et al., 2024).

Synthetic fragrance chemicals are produced through industrial chemical processes, frequently using petroleum-derived feedstocks. These compounds are favored in commercial manufacturing due to cost efficiency, consistency, and enhanced longevity. Synthetic musks (e.g., galaxolide, tonalide) and phthalates are common examples of fragrance chemicals designed to persist on skin and fabric and resist degradation (Reiner et al., 2007). Emerging concerns include nanotechnology in some synthetic formulations, which may enable deeper penetration and greater toxicity risks, including oxidative stress and inflammation (Johnson, 2025). Studies associate synthetic fragrances with allergies, respiratory issues, endocrine disruption, reproductive problems, and potential cancer risks (Ahmed et al., 2024; Martins et al., 2023).

Fragrance and Ingredient Disclosure Loopholes

Trade secret protections allow fragrance ingredients to be exempt from full disclosure requirements. This exemption applies even when fragrance chemicals include substances associated with endocrine disruption, respiratory irritation, or sensitization (Steinemann, 2016). Products labeled as fragrance-free may still contain masking fragrances used to suppress odor, while unscented products often include fragrance compounds for the same purpose. Consumer surveys demonstrate that most individuals are unaware of these labeling practices, leading to unintentional exposure even among those actively attempting to avoid fragrance (Steinemann, 2018). Ongoing U.S. FDA proposals and state-level expansions (e.g., California) reflect growing pressure for greater transparency on allergens (FDA Unified Regulatory Agenda, 2025).

Volatility and Indoor Air Chemistry

Fragrance chemicals are intentionally designed to volatilize, meaning they readily evaporate at room temperature and disperse into indoor air. Once airborne, these compounds are inhaled and absorbed through the respiratory tract. Studies show that fragrance-derived terpenes such as limonene and alpha-pinene react with indoor ozone to form secondary pollutants, including formaldehyde and ultrafine particulate matter (Weschler & Shields, 1997; Nazaroff & Weschler, 2004). Recent research (2024–2025) demonstrates that these reactions produce nanoparticles at concentrations rivaling combustion sources like gas stoves, penetrating deep into the lungs and contributing to oxidative stress, inflammation, and airway irritation (Jung et al., 2025; Purdue University, 2025; Katam et al., 2025). Scented wax melts and non-combustion products release high terpene levels, amplifying nanoparticle formation indoors (ACS ES&T Letters, 2025).

Chemical Fixatives and Prolonged Exposure: Why Lingering Scents Matter

Chemical fixatives are substances added to fragranced products to make scents last longer by slowing evaporation and stabilizing volatile fragrance compounds. While this may enhance product appeal, it also prolongs human exposure to airborne chemicals. Fixatives allow fragrance compounds to linger in indoor air, settle on surfaces, and remain on skin and clothing for extended periods of time. This extended exposure increases the likelihood of inhalation and absorption, particularly in enclosed environments such as homes, workplaces, and healthcare settings. For sensitive individuals, prolonged exposure to fixatives can intensify symptoms such as headaches, respiratory irritation, dizziness, and allergic reactions. Over time, repeated exposure may contribute to chronic inflammatory responses and cumulative toxic burden, raising legitimate concerns about the health impact of fragranced products that rely on chemical fixatives to sustain scent persistence.

Common chemical fixatives used in fragranced products include phthalates such as diethyl phthalate (DEP), which are added to stabilize scent and slow evaporation. Synthetic musks like galaxolide and tonalide are also widely used fixatives that help fragrances persist on skin and in indoor air. Other examples include benzyl benzoate, benzyl salicylate, and triethyl citrate, which anchor volatile fragrance compounds and extend their longevity. While effective at making scents last, these fixatives increase the duration of chemical exposure and have been associated with respiratory irritation, headaches, allergic reactions, and concerns related to hormone disruption and cumulative toxic burden in sensitive individuals.

Lipophilicity and Bioaccumulation

Many fragrance compounds are lipophilic, meaning they dissolve readily in fat. This property facilitates dermal absorption and systemic distribution. Bioaccumulative fragrance chemicals, including synthetic musks, have been detected in human adipose tissue, breast milk, and umbilical cord blood, indicating chronic exposure and transgenerational transfer potential (Reiner et al., 2007; Luo et al., 2023). Recent environmental monitoring confirms widespread occurrence of synthetic musks in aquatic and human tissues, with persistence and potential for enhanced toxicity from transformation products (Luo et al., 2023). Phthalates, common fixatives, contribute to bioaccumulation and endocrine disruption (Ahmed et al., 2024).

Mixture Toxicity and Real-World Exposure

Toxicological testing typically evaluates single chemicals in isolation. Fragrance exposure occurs as a mixture. Individuals are exposed to complex chemical combinations from personal care products, household cleaners, laundry products, and fragranced public spaces. Research on chemical mixtures indicates that combined exposures can produce additive or synergistic effects, even when individual components are present at levels considered safe in isolation (Kortenkamp & Faust, 2018; Martins et al., 2023). Synergistic interactions may amplify endocrine disruption, respiratory irritation, or other effects in real-world scenarios (Ahmed et al., 2024).

Synthetic Musks: Persistent Fragrance Chemicals

Synthetic musks are laboratory-manufactured fragrance compounds used to create and stabilize "musky" scent profiles in perfumes, personal care products, cleaning agents, detergents, air fresheners, and cosmetics. Because natural animal-derived musk became ethically restricted and commercially impractical, synthetic alternatives were developed and widely adopted throughout the twentieth century. Today, synthetic musks are among the most commonly used fragrance ingredients globally. Unlike many volatile fragrance components that dissipate quickly, synthetic musks are intentionally engineered to persist. Their chemical stability, lipophilicity, and resistance to degradation allow them to remain in products, indoor air, household dust, waterways, and human tissues. These characteristics raise important toxicological and public health concerns.

Classes of Synthetic Musks

Synthetic musks are generally divided into three major categories.

- **Nitro musks** were among the earliest synthetic variants. Compounds such as musk xylene and musk ketone were widely used in the mid-twentieth century. Due to concerns about environmental persistence, bioaccumulation, and potential toxicological effects, several nitro musks have been restricted or phased out in parts of Europe and other regions (European Chemicals Agency, 2010).
- **Polycyclic musks**, including galaxolide (HHCB) and tonalide (AHTN), replaced nitro musks and remain common in modern consumer products. These compounds are highly persistent and have been detected in surface water, sediment, household dust, human adipose tissue, and breast milk (Bester, 2009; Reiner & Kannan, 2006). Their widespread detection reflects both environmental stability and continuous human exposure.
- **Macrocyclic musks** represent a newer generation of fragrance compounds marketed as safer alternatives. While they are considered less bioaccumulative than earlier classes, long-term independent human health data remain limited.

Vulnerable Populations

Certain populations are particularly susceptible to fragrance exposure. Children, pregnant individuals, and those with asthma, migraines, autoimmune conditions, or chemical sensitivities demonstrate heightened vulnerability in clinical and epidemiological studies (Caress & Steinemann, 2009). Occupational exposure further increases risk for healthcare workers, educators, service industry employees, and salon professionals.

Why Understanding Fragrance Matters

Fragrance is not a passive cosmetic feature. It is an active chemical system designed to interact with human sensory pathways and the indoor environment. Because exposure is widespread, repeated, and largely invisible, fragrance-related illness is frequently misattributed to stress, allergy, or psychological factors. Understanding what fragrance is reframes these symptoms as biologically supported responses to chemical exposure. This awareness is foundational for recognizing health effects discussed in later chapters, including hormonal disruption, respiratory disease, neurological symptoms, immune activation, and long-term toxic burden.

Conclusion

Fragrance is not a single ingredient but a complex, undisclosed chemical mixture engineered for persistence and exposure. Understanding fragrance composition, volatility, and bioaccumulation clarifies why adverse health effects occur and why consumer awareness remains limited. Transparency is essential for informed health decisions.

FAQ

Frequently Asked Questions: Fragrance and Health

Is fragrance sensitivity the same as an allergy?

No. Fragrance sensitivity is not the same as a classic IgE-mediated allergy. While some individuals may have allergic contact dermatitis or respiratory allergies to specific compounds, most fragrance reactions occur through non–IgE-mediated mechanisms, including neurological sensitization, immune activation, irritant responses, and inflammatory signaling (Caress & Steinemann, 2009). This distinction explains why standard allergy testing (e.g., skin prick or IgE blood tests) often fails to identify the cause of symptoms despite clear and reproducible reactions. Respiratory symptoms are frequently irritant-based rather than true allergic (Verywell Health, 2025; Allergic Living, 2014).

Why do my symptoms feel neurological rather than respiratory?

Fragrance chemicals are readily absorbed through the lungs and can cross the blood–brain barrier, allowing direct interaction with the central nervous system (Doty, 2001). The **olfactory system** is the body's sensory pathway responsible for detecting odors. When a scent is inhaled, odor molecules travel through the

Olfactory System & Limbic System Response to Toxic Fragrance

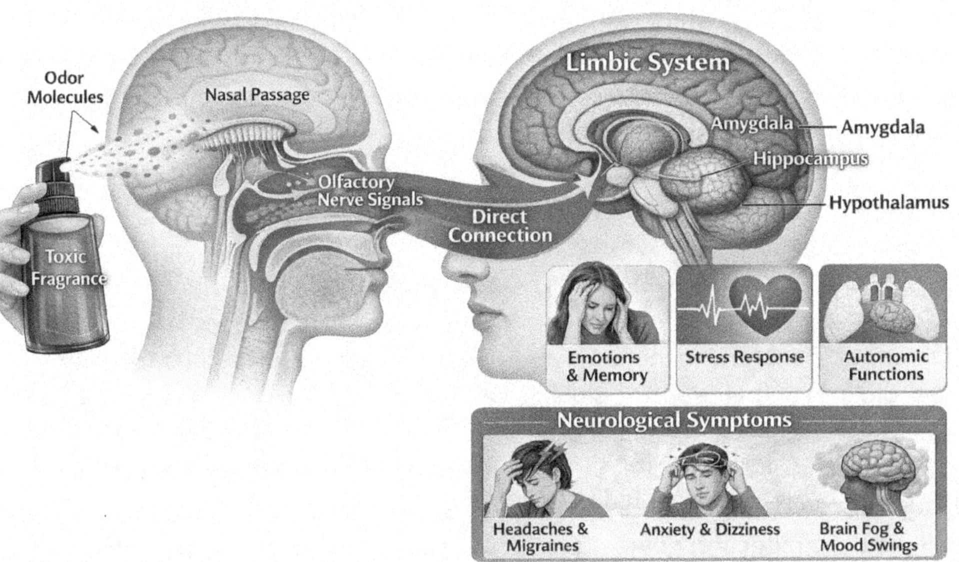

nasal passages and bind to specialized receptors that send signals directly to the brain. Unlike other sensory systems, the olfactory system bypasses many filtering and processing pathways and delivers information rapidly.

The **limbic system** is a group of interconnected brain structures that regulate emotions, memory, stress responses, and involuntary body functions such as heart rate and breathing. Because the olfactory system connects directly to the limbic system, inhaled chemicals can quickly influence emotional and neurological regulation. This direct connection explains why exposure to fragranced chemicals can trigger neurological symptoms such as headaches, migraines, dizziness, anxiety, confusion, cognitive fog, or sudden mood changes. In many individuals, these neurological effects occur before or even without obvious respiratory symptoms, particularly after central sensitization has developed, when the nervous system becomes hyperresponsive to repeated exposures (Woolf, 2011; Martins et al., 2023).

Why did I tolerate fragrance for years and then suddenly become sensitive?

Tolerance to chemical exposure is not permanent. Over time, repeated exposure increases cumulative toxic burden while reducing physiological resilience through mechanisms like immune dysregulation and nervous system sensitization. Triggers such as illness, chronic stress, hormonal changes, mold exposure, pregnancy, surgery, or other environmental insults can overwhelm detoxification and regulatory systems, leading to loss of tolerance (Landrigan et al., 2018). Once this threshold is crossed, even low-level exposures can provoke disproportionate responses (Steinemann, 2016).

Can fragrance sensitivity get worse with continued exposure?

Yes. Continued exposure reinforces neurological sensitization, a process in which the nervous system becomes increasingly hypersensitive to repeated stimuli. With ongoing exposure, the brain and peripheral nerves lower their reaction threshold and amplify sensory signals, causing the body to respond more quickly and intensely to even minimal triggers. This heightened state perpetuates inflammatory signaling and dysregulation across multiple systems. Over time, symptoms can become more frequent, more severe, longer lasting, and multisystemic, affecting neurological, respiratory, cardiovascular, and immune function (Woolf, 2011). For many individuals, strict avoidance of triggering exposures is necessary to interrupt this cycle, reduce nervous system overactivation, and allow meaningful recovery to occur.

Why do my symptoms sometimes start hours or days after exposure?

Delayed reactions are common and stem from immune signaling, endocrine disruption, and inflammatory cascades rather than immediate irritation. Fragrance chemicals can alter hormone pathways and trigger systemic inflammation that unfolds gradually, leading to delayed fatigue, migraines, mood changes, or other symptoms (Diamanti-Kandarakis et al., 2009). These are often misattributed to unrelated causes.

Is this condition psychological or anxiety-driven?

No. While anxiety can amplify physiological symptoms, it does not cause fragrance sensitivity. Neurogenic inflammation, immune activation, central nervous system sensitization, and irritant responses are well-documented biological processes triggered by chemical exposure (Meggs, 1995). Dismissing symptoms as psychological overlooks the underlying pathophysiology and delays effective intervention (Steinemann, 2016).

Why do some people react strongly while others seem unaffected?

Individual susceptibility varies widely due to genetics, prior toxic exposures, immune function, nervous system regulation, hormonal status, total inflammatory load, and comorbidities. Higher prevalence occurs in those with asthma (up to 60–75%), chemical sensitivity, or autism spectrum disorders (Steinemann et al., 2019; Steinemann, 2021). The lack of symptoms in others does not indicate universal safety.

Can fragrance exposure worsen existing medical conditions?

Yes. Fragrance exposure exacerbates asthma, migraines, autoimmune conditions, chronic pain syndromes, neuroinflammatory disorders, sinus issues, and fatigue (Anderson & Anderson, 1998; Miller et al., 2007). It can also intensify cognitive impairment, mood instability, and respiratory symptoms in vulnerable groups (Ohio State Health & Discovery, 2023).

Does "natural" or "essential oil–based" fragrance make products safe?

No. Natural origin does not guarantee safety. Essential oils and botanical extracts contain potent volatile compounds (e.g., limonene, linalool) that can trigger neurological, immune, respiratory, or allergic reactions, often comparable to synthetics (de Groot, 2021; Ahmed et al., 2024). Recent studies link prolonged essential oil inhalation to cardiopulmonary effects, endocrine disruption, and increased risks in sensitive individuals (American Lung Association, 2024; NIEHS, ongoing).

Why do "fragrance-free" or "unscented" products still cause reactions?

"Fragrance-free" does not mean irritant-free. Manufacturers may add masking agents (which are fragrances) to neutralize chemical odors, or include undisclosed botanicals, preservatives, or essential oil derivatives that trigger sensitivities. "Unscented" products often use these masking fragrances. True avoidance requires checking full ingredient lists and patch testing (Pure Haven, 2024; Clinikally, 2025).

Is fragrance sensitivity related to multiple chemical sensitivity (MCS)?

Yes, often. Many with fragrance sensitivity develop or experience broader MCS, reacting to low levels of various chemicals (e.g., cleaning agents, exhaust, plastics). Fragrances are a major trigger for MCS symptoms like headaches, fatigue, and respiratory issues, affecting up to 1–4% of populations in some studies (ASEQ-EHAQ, 2024; ILRU.org).

Are children, pregnant people, or the elderly at higher risk?

Yes. Vulnerable groups face amplified risks due to developing or declining detoxification systems. Prenatal exposure to phthalates/fragrance chemicals links to developmental delays, asthma, behavioral issues, and reproductive harm in children. Children absorb more per body weight; elderly may have reduced resilience; pregnant individuals risk endocrine disruption and fetal effects (UC Davis Health, 2025; Harvard Health, 2019; PMC review, 2024).

How can I get accommodations at work or school?

Fragrance sensitivity qualifies as a disability under laws like the ADA (U.S.) or similar frameworks elsewhere. Reasonable accommodations include scent-free policies, ventilation improvements, or remote options. Documentation from a healthcare provider strengthens requests (Job Accommodation Network; ScienceDirect, 2019).

What is the most important step for recovery?

The most critical step is comprehensive exposure reduction across personal care, laundry, cleaning, indoor air, and shared spaces. Without minimizing triggers, supportive therapies (e.g., nervous system stabilization) are limited. Environmental control is foundational for symptom stabilization and healing (Steinemann, 2016).

Biological Mechanisms and Common Questions

Fragrance sensitivity is a genuine physical response in the body, not something imagined, psychological, or related to personality. It is caused by chemical compounds in synthetic fragrances that affect the brain, immune system, hormonal pathways, and other biological systems, particularly with repeated exposure over time (Steinemann, 2016). Understanding how these chemicals interact with the body helps explain why symptoms often worsen rather than improve, and why individuals who were once unaffected by scents may suddenly begin experiencing significant and debilitating reactions.

What "Fragrance" Really Means

"Fragrance" or "perfume" on a label does not refer to a single ingredient. It represents a concealed mixture of dozens or even hundreds of chemicals. Many of these substances are volatile organic compounds, which are small particles that easily become airborne. Manufacturers are not required to disclose all fragrance components because of trade secret protections, even though some of these chemicals are known to irritate the lungs, affect the nervous system, or disrupt hormonal balance (Steinemann et al., 2011). These chemicals are released into the air from perfumes, soaps, cleaning products, laundry detergents, candles, air fresheners, and similar items. They are inhaled daily, enter the bloodstream rapidly, and in some cases can reach the brain directly.

How Scents Affect Your Brain and Nerves (Neurological Sensitization)

Your nose connects straight to the limbic system, a part of the brain that regulates emotions, memory, stress, and automatic body functions such as heart rate. Smells bypass the brain's usual filtering pathways and reach this area very quickly. This is why a scent can immediately trigger anxiety, dizziness, or a headache (Herz, 2009). With repeated exposure to irritating fragrance chemicals,

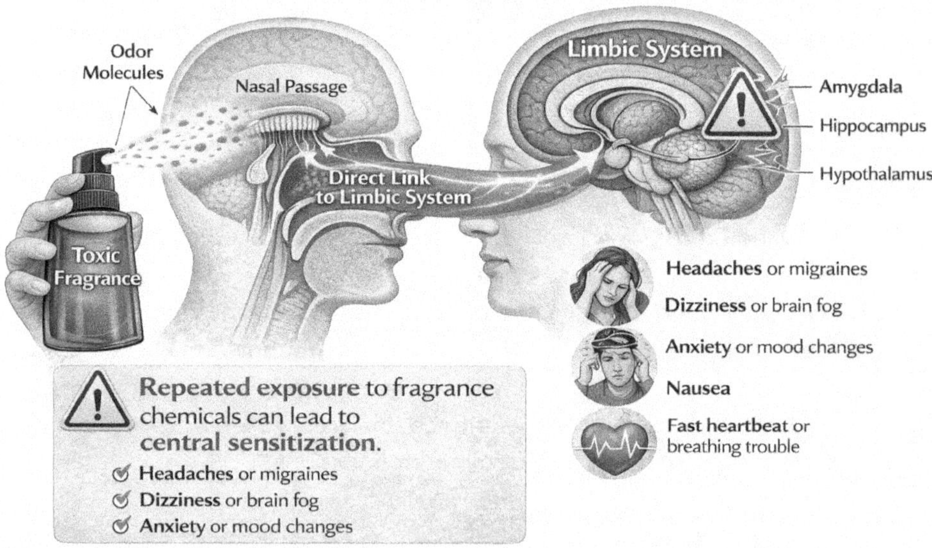

the nervous system can become overly sensitive, a process known as central sensitization. In this state, the body's alarm system is essentially turned up, so small amounts of scent that were once tolerated can provoke intense reactions (Woolf, 2011). This can cause:

- Headaches or migraines
- Dizziness or brain fog
- Anxiety or mood changes
- Nausea
- Fast heartbeat or breathing trouble

In people with this sensitivity, the brain treats the scent like a threat, even if it's harmless.

Immune System Reactions and Inflammation

Your body sees some fragrance chemicals as invaders. It can trigger immune responses that aren't the classic "allergy" type (no positive skin prick test), but still cause inflammation (Caress & Steinemann, 2009). This releases chemicals like cytokines and histamine, which spread through the body and cause:

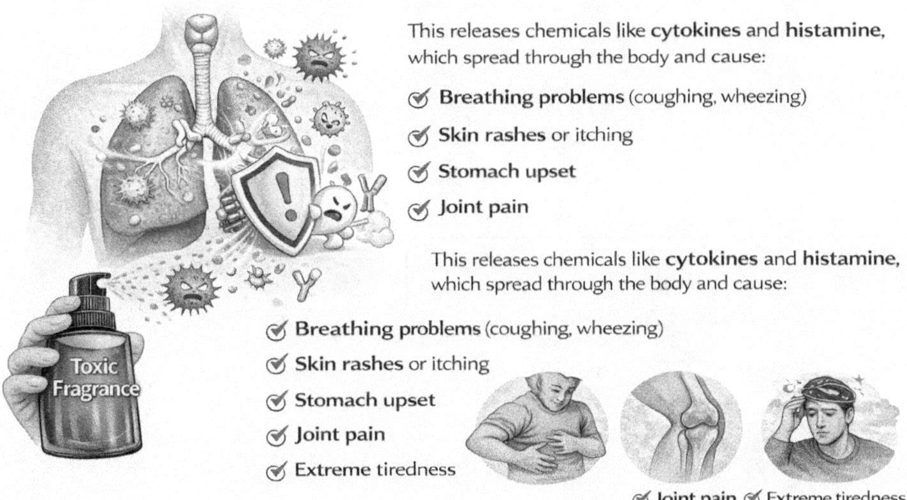

- Breathing problems (coughing, wheezing)
- Skin rashes or itching

- Stomach upset
- Joint pain
- Extreme tiredness

These reactions can affect many body parts at once and often don't show up on standard allergy tests, so doctors might think it's "just stress." But it's real inflammation (Anderson & Anderson, 1998; Macchione et al., 2024).

Hormone Disruption (Endocrine Effects)

Many fragrance chemicals act as hormone mimics or interfere with normal hormonal signaling in the body. Common examples include phthalates, which are used to make scents last longer, and synthetic musks. These substances can disrupt estrogen, testosterone, thyroid, and stress hormone pathways, even at very low levels of exposure (Diamanti-Kandarakis et al., 2009). This helps explain:

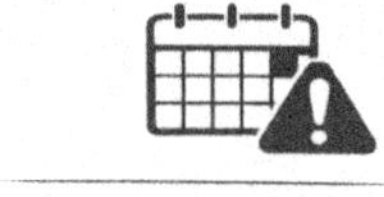

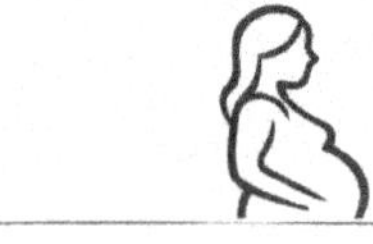

- Irregular periods or fertility issues
- Thyroid problems

- Mood swings or fatigue
- Symptoms that get worse during pregnancy, puberty, or menopause

Effects can show up hours or days later as hormones get out of balance. Recent studies link these chemicals to early puberty in girls, reproductive harm, and higher risks of certain cancers (Ahmed et al., 2024; EWG, 2024; NIH, 2024).

Why It Builds Up Over Time (Cumulative Toxic Load)

Your body has ways to break down and remove toxins (like through the liver and kidneys). But daily exposure from many products adds up, storing some chemicals in fat and brain tissue. Over years, this "toxic load" can overwhelm your system. Then symptoms start (Landrigan et al., 2018).

What Causes It to Begin or Get Worse?

Many people point to a specific event before symptoms began or got bad, like:

- A bad virus or illness
- Mold in the home
- Surgery or anesthesia
- Pregnancy or hormone changes
- High stress
- Heavy exposure to chemicals (e.g., pesticides)

These events stress the body, making it harder to handle scents it once ignored (Miller et al., 2007).

Why Symptoms Differ from Person to Person

Not everyone reacts the same way. It depends on genes, past exposures, immune health, hormone levels, and overall body stress. Some get mostly breathing issues; others get brain fog or pain. No symptoms in someone else doesn't mean it's safe for you.

Why People Say "It's All in Your Head"—and Why That's Wrong

Symptoms are often called psychological because they're hard to test and invisible. But brain scans and studies show real changes in nerve signals and immune activity from chemical exposure (Meggs, 1995). Stress can make things feel worse, but it doesn't cause the problem.

Why Avoiding Scents Is So Important

Once the nervous system becomes sensitized, continued exposure repeatedly irritates nerves and sustains inflammation. Reducing or eliminating exposure allows the body to settle and begin recovery. In this context, avoidance is not optional; it is the primary and most effective treatment.

Final Note

Fragrance sensitivity reflects real biological injury involving the nervous, immune, endocrine, and respiratory systems. These reactions are predictable, reproducible, and supported by scientific evidence. Understanding mechanisms, reducing exposure, and seeking informed care are essential for prevention, management, and recovery.

Poison by Design

Synthetic fragrance chemicals are not accidental contaminants. They are intentionally engineered substances designed to disperse efficiently, persist in the environment, adhere to surfaces, and interact with human sensory and biological systems. **The health risks associated with fragrance exposure are <u>not the result of misuse</u> but rather the predictable outcome of chemical design choices made to maximize scent longevity, diffusion, and commercial appeal.**

Engineering for Persistence and Penetration

Fragrance compounds are selected based on their volatility, stability, and ability to bind to materials such as skin, hair, fabric, and indoor surfaces. Many fragrance chemicals are semi-volatile organic compounds that do not evaporate immediately but continue to off-gas over time, extending exposure well beyond initial application (Weschler, 2009). Lipophilic properties are central to fragrance design. Lipophilic chemicals readily dissolve in fat, allowing them to penetrate the skin barrier, cross biological membranes, and accumulate in adipose tissue. This property increases systemic exposure and contributes to bioaccumulation with repeated daily use (Reiner et al., 2007). Recent reviews confirm that synthetic musks and phthalates exhibit high persistence and bioaccumulative potential, leading to detection in human tissues, breast milk, and umbilical cord blood, with concerns for chronic hormonal disruption and developmental effects (Luo et al., 2023; Ashcroft et al., 2024).

Volatile Organic Compounds (VOC) and Toxic Load

Analytical studies have identified dozens to hundreds of volatile organic compounds emitted from fragranced products, many of which are classified as hazardous air pollutants under United States federal regulations (Steinemann, 2011). These include benzene derivatives, aldehydes, and terpenes that contribute to respiratory irritation, oxidative stress, and neurological symptoms. Indoor exposure is particularly concerning because fragrance chemicals are released into enclosed environments where ventilation is limited. Once airborne, these compounds are inhaled directly into the lungs, bypassing hepatic detoxification pathways and allowing rapid systemic distribution (Nazaroff & Weschler, 2004). Recent analyses show that even "green" or fragrance-free labeled products can emit similar hazardous VOC profiles (Steinemann, 2015).

Secondary Pollutant Formation

Fragrance chemicals do not remain chemically inert once released. Terpenes such as limonene and alpha-pinene react with indoor ozone to form secondary pollutants, including formaldehyde, acetaldehyde, and ultrafine particulate matter (Weschler & Shields, 1997). These secondary compounds often exhibit greater toxicity than the original fragrance ingredients. Studies have linked secondary indoor pollutants to airway inflammation, epithelial damage, and increased asthma symptoms. Importantly, these reactions occur at common indoor ozone concentrations, meaning exposure can occur in ordinary household and workplace environments (Weschler, 2006). Recent chamber studies demonstrate rapid new particle formation from fragranced personal care products reacting with ozone, with particle growth rates far exceeding typical outdoor events and leading to high concentrations of ultrafine particles and oxygenated VOCs (Jung et al., 2025; Katam et al., 2025).

Endocrine Active Design Features

Many fragrance chemicals are deliberately designed to resist degradation. Phthalates, commonly used as fragrance fixatives, slow evaporation and prolong scent persistence. These compounds are now well established as endocrine disrupting chemicals with estrogenic and antiandrogenic activity (Meeker et al., 2009). Synthetic musks are another example of toxic design. These compounds are engineered to be stable and long lasting, yet they demonstrate bioaccumulative properties and have been detected in human tissue, breast milk, and umbilical cord blood (Reiner et al., 2007). Their persistence raises concerns regarding chronic hormonal disruption and developmental exposure. Recent reviews highlight synthetic musks and phthalates as endocrine disruptors affecting thyroid, androgen, and estrogen pathways, linking to reproductive toxicity, cancer risks, and metabolic disorders (Kim & Park, 2023; Ashcroft et al., 2024; Ahmed et al., 2024).

Mixture Toxicity and Synergistic Effects

Fragrance exposure rarely occurs in isolation. Individuals are exposed to complex chemical mixtures from multiple fragranced products used throughout the day. Toxicological studies increasingly demonstrate that chemical mixtures can exert additive or synergistic effects even when individual components are present at levels deemed safe in isolation (Kortenkamp & Faust, 2018). Traditional safety assessments do not adequately account for cumulative exposure, mixture toxicity, or vulnerable populations. This gap creates a false sense of safety that does not reflect real world conditions. Recent narrative reviews emphasize that combined exposures from personal care and household products amplify risks, including endocrine-immune-neural axis perturbation (Martins et al., 2023).

Regulatory Gaps and Safety Assumptions

Fragrance ingredients are often classified as safe based on limited testing that does not reflect chronic exposure, inhalation pathways, or combined chemical effects. Regulatory frameworks frequently rely on industry supplied data and self regulation through trade associations rather than independent long term safety evaluation (Steinemann, 2016). The phrase safe as used does not account for repeated daily exposure beginning in infancy, nor does it consider individuals with asthma, migraines, autoimmune disease, or chemical sensitivity. This regulatory approach prioritizes commercial interests over precautionary public health principles.

Occupational and High Dose Exposure

Occupational settings amplify exposure risks. Healthcare workers, salon professionals, cleaners, educators, and service industry employees are often exposed to fragranced products for extended periods in enclosed spaces. Studies demonstrate higher prevalence of respiratory symptoms, headaches, and neurological complaints among workers in fragranced environments (Caress & Steinemann, 2009). In these settings, fragrance exposure is not optional. This raises ethical and occupational health concerns, particularly when safer alternatives are readily available. Recent research in beauty salons identifies elevated VOCs and carbonyls, with hazard quotients for formaldehyde and acetaldehyde exceeding acceptable levels, and increased reports of dry eyes, skin irritation, and respiratory issues among technicians (Kim et al., 2023).

Predictable Harm

The health effects associated with synthetic fragrance exposure are not random or rare. They are the predictable result of chemical properties intentionally selected to enhance persistence, diffusion, and consumer appeal. When compounds are designed to linger in air, bind to tissue, resist breakdown, and evade disclosure, biological consequences should be expected.

Poison by design does not imply malicious intent. It reflects a system in which chemical performance is prioritized over biological compatibility. The result is widespread, chronic exposure to substances capable of disrupting respiratory, neurological, endocrine, and immune function. Understanding this design framework is essential for recognizing why fragrance exposure produces consistent health effects across diverse populations. It also underscores the need for transparency, regulation reform, and informed consumer choice, which will be explored in subsequent chapters.

Conclusion

The health effects of fragrance exposure are predictable consequences of chemical design choices that prioritize longevity, diffusion, and stability. When compounds are engineered to persist, bind to tissue, and resist degradation, biological consequences are inevitable. This design framework demands reevaluation of safety assumptions and regulatory standards.

The Invisible Exposure

Synthetic fragrance exposure is largely invisible, yet it represents one of the most persistent and unavoidable chemical contacts in modern life. Unlike industrial pollutants that are clearly identified as hazards, fragrance exposure is normalized, socially reinforced, and rarely recognized as a source of illness. This invisibility does not reflect low exposure. It reflects how fragrance chemicals behave in the environment and how their risks are framed.

Ubiquity of Fragranced Products

Fragranced products are present in nearly every indoor environment. Personal care items, cleaning agents, laundry products, air fresheners, scented candles, and fragranced building materials continuously introduce fragrance chemicals into indoor air. Studies show that most individuals are exposed to multiple fragranced products each day, often without awareness (Steinemann, 2018). Importantly, exposure is frequently involuntary. Population studies demonstrate that many individuals report health effects from fragranced products used by others in shared environments such as workplaces, schools, healthcare facilities, public transportation, and retail spaces (Steinemann et al., 2016). This involuntary exposure significantly increases cumulative toxic burden.

Airborne Exposure Pathways

Fragrance chemicals are engineered to volatilize. Once released, they disperse into indoor air and are inhaled directly into the respiratory tract. Inhaled chemicals bypass first pass metabolism by the liver, allowing rapid systemic distribution. Even low concentration airborne exposures can be biologically significant due to repeated and prolonged inhalation (Nazaroff & Weschler, 2004). Indoor air quality studies consistently identify fragranced products as a major source of volatile organic compounds. Elevated concentrations persist for hours to days depending on ventilation and chemical composition (Weschler, 2009).

Surface Binding and Secondary Exposure

Fragrance chemicals do not remain airborne indefinitely. Many bind to surfaces including walls, furniture, carpets, clothing, and skin. Once bound, these compounds continue to off gas over time, creating ongoing secondary exposure even after the original product application has ended (Steinemann, 2011). Laundry products are particularly effective at embedding fragrance chemicals into fabrics. This creates continuous exposure through inhalation and direct skin contact, often lasting for days or weeks.

Dermal Absorption Through Skin Contact

Skin contact represents a major and underrecognized exposure pathway for fragrance chemicals. Human skin is not an impermeable barrier. Many fragrance compounds are lipophilic and readily penetrate the stratum corneum, allowing systemic absorption. Experimental and modeling studies indicate that dermal absorption of fragrance chemicals can range widely depending on chemical properties, concentration, formulation, and duration of contact. For many fragrance ingredients, estimated dermal absorption ranges from approximately 10 percent to more than 60 percent of the applied dose (Brown et al., 2013; WHO, 2011). Highly lipophilic compounds such as synthetic musks and certain phthalates demonstrate particularly efficient skin penetration and systemic uptake (Api et al., 2015).

Regulatory assessments by the European Commission and World Health Organization acknowledge that dermal exposure from fragranced personal care products often represents the dominant exposure route, exceeding inhalation exposure for many compounds due to prolonged skin contact and repeated daily use (WHO, 2011; SCCS, 2012). Once absorbed, fragrance chemicals can enter systemic circulation, accumulate in adipose tissue, and persist due to slow metabolic clearance. Detection of fragrance compounds in human blood, breast milk, and adipose tissue confirms that dermal exposure contributes meaningfully to internal chemical load (Reiner et al., 2007).

Misattribution of Symptoms

Because fragrance exposure is socially normalized, symptoms triggered by synthetic scents are frequently misattributed. Headaches, fatigue, respiratory irritation, dizziness, nausea, cognitive impairment, and mood changes are often labeled as stress, allergy, anxiety, or idiopathic illness. Clinical case studies document symptom improvement or resolution following fragrance avoidance, supporting a causal relationship that is commonly overlooked (Ziem & McTamney, 1997). This misattribution delays recognition, prolongs exposure, and reinforces the false belief that fragrance related illness reflects individual sensitivity rather than predictable toxicological response.

Vulnerable Populations and Silent Risk

Certain populations face disproportionate risk. Children absorb higher relative doses due to greater surface area to body weight ratio and higher respiratory rates. Pregnant individuals may transfer lipophilic fragrance chemicals across the placenta. Individuals with asthma, migraines, autoimmune disease, or chemical sensitivity demonstrate heightened vulnerability in epidemiological studies (Caress & Steinemann, 2009). Occupational exposure further amplifies risk. Healthcare workers, educators, service industry employees, and salon professionals often experience continuous exposure in enclosed spaces. Studies consistently report higher prevalence of respiratory and neurological symptoms in these populations, yet fragrance exposure remains largely unrecognized as an occupational hazard (Steinemann, 2018).

Social Normalization and Invisibility

Fragrance persists in part due to cultural norms that associate scent with cleanliness, professionalism, and social acceptability. These norms discourage individuals from questioning exposure or requesting fragrance free environments. Surveys indicate that affected individuals frequently avoid public spaces rather than request accommodation, reinforcing invisibility and isolation (Steinemann et al., 2016).

The Cumulative Burden

Invisible exposure becomes most harmful through accumulation. Daily contact with multiple fragranced products results in continuous low dose exposure across inhalation and dermal pathways. Chemical mixtures interact within the body and environment, compounding toxic burden over time. Traditional safety assessments do not adequately account for this cumulative reality (Kortenkamp & Faust, 2018).

Making the Invisible Visible

Synthetic fragrance exposure is not rare or minor. It is a predictable consequence of widespread chemical use combined with limited disclosure and weak regulatory oversight. Recognizing fragrance as an invisible exposure source is essential for understanding chronic symptoms, unexplained illness, and environmental health disparities. By making the invisible visible, individuals and institutions can begin to identify exposure sources, reduce unnecessary contact, and protect vulnerable populations. The chapters that follow examine how this exposure affects specific body systems, beginning with the nervous system and hormonal regulation.

Conclusion

Fragrance exposure is ubiquitous, often involuntary, and cumulative. Airborne dispersion, surface adhesion, and dermal absorption result in continuous exposure that is frequently misattributed or overlooked. Making this invisible exposure visible is essential to reducing toxic burden and protecting vulnerable populations.

Occupational Exposure

For many individuals, the greatest exposure to synthetic fragrance does not occur at home. It occurs in the workplace. Occupational environments often involve prolonged, repeated, and unavoidable exposure, making them a major contributor to cumulative chemical burden. Because exposure is frequent and often outside individual control, occupational fragrance exposure carries distinct health risks.

Occupational Exposure Intensity

Occupational exposure is defined by three factors: concentration, duration, and frequency. Workers may be exposed for eight to twelve hours per day, five or more days per week, often in enclosed environments with limited ventilation. This pattern significantly amplifies risk compared to intermittent household exposure. Population studies consistently demonstrate that occupational fragrance exposure produces higher symptom prevalence than general consumer exposure.

Overall Health Impact of Workplace Fragrance Exposure

Large scale surveys conducted in the United States, Australia, and Europe report that approximately **20 to 34 percent of adults** experience adverse health effects from fragranced products in public or occupational settings (Steinemann, 2016; 2018). Among those affected, workplace exposure accounts for a substantial proportion of reported symptoms due to duration and intensity. Reported effects include headaches, migraines, respiratory distress, asthma exacerbation, neurological symptoms, skin reactions, and cognitive impairment.

Healthcare and Caregiving Professions

Exposure intensity: High
Duration: Long shifts, enclosed spaces
Control: Low
Healthcare workers are routinely exposed to fragranced cleaning agents, soaps, sanitizers, personal care products, and laundry chemicals.
Studies show that **over 30 percent of healthcare workers** report fragrance related health symptoms, including headaches, respiratory irritation, dizziness, and nausea (Steinemann, 2018). Asthma exacerbation is particularly common.

Fragranced product exposure is a recognized trigger for work related asthma, with healthcare workers representing a high risk group due to repeated exposure (Caress & Steinemann, 2009).

Education and Childcare Settings

Exposure intensity: Moderate to high
Duration: Full workday
Control: Low to moderate
Teachers and childcare workers are exposed through cleaning products, air fresheners, scented classroom supplies, and personal fragrances worn by others. Research indicates that **over 25 percent of teachers** report headaches or respiratory symptoms linked to fragranced products in school environments (Mendell, 2004). Children are also exposed in these settings, compounding concern due to developmental vulnerability.

Salon, Beauty, and Personal Service Industries

Exposure intensity: Very high
Duration: Continuous
Control: Minimal
Salon workers experience some of the highest occupational fragrance exposures due to constant inhalation of scented sprays, aerosols, hair products, and cosmetics, as well as direct skin contact. Studies report that **40 to 60 percent of salon workers** experience respiratory symptoms, headaches, dermatitis, or neurological complaints associated with chemical exposure (Quach et al., 2011). Chronic exposure in these settings has been associated with endocrine disruption and reproductive effects, particularly among women of reproductive age.

Hospitality, Retail, and Service Industries
Exposure intensity: Moderate to high
Duration: Long shifts
Control: Low
Hotels, retail stores, gyms, and restaurants frequently use fragranced cleaning agents and ambient scent marketing systems. Surveys show that **over 20 percent of workers** in fragranced retail and service environments report adverse

health effects, and a significant subset report reduced work performance or missed workdays due to symptoms (Steinemann, 2016). Scent marketing increases airborne fragrance concentration deliberately, intensifying exposure beyond personal product use.

Manufacturing and Industrial Settings

Exposure intensity: High to extreme
Duration: Prolonged
Control: Variable
Workers involved in fragrance production, chemical manufacturing, packaging, or transport may encounter concentrated fragrance compounds. While occupational safety standards exist, ingredient disclosure is limited due to trade secret protections. This restricts comprehensive exposure assessment and risk evaluation. These workers experience higher risk for respiratory irritation, neurological symptoms, and sensitization due to concentrated exposure.

Symptom Severity and Cumulative Risk

Repeated occupational exposure lowers symptom thresholds over time. Individuals may develop increased sensitivity, meaning lower levels of fragrance trigger stronger reactions.

Reported outcomes include:

- Chronic headaches and migraines
- Work related asthma and respiratory distress
- Cognitive impairment and concentration difficulty
- Skin irritation and dermatitis
- Fatigue and neurological symptoms

In population studies, **over 10 percent of affected individuals** report that fragrance exposure is disabling enough to restrict daily activities or employment (Steinemann, 2018).

Vulnerable Worker Populations

Pregnant workers, individuals with asthma, migraines, autoimmune disease, neurological disorders, or prior chemical sensitivity face increased risk. Because fragrance exposure is often normalized, many workers remain exposed despite worsening symptoms, fearing stigma or job insecurity.

Fragrance Free Workplace Policies

Evidence demonstrates that fragrance free workplace policies reduce symptom prevalence and improve productivity without compromising cleanliness or professionalism. In surveys, **over 50 percent of workers** support fragrance free policies when informed of health impacts, indicating strong acceptability when framed as a health and safety issue (Steinemann, 2016).

Worker Advocacy and Protection

Workers experiencing symptoms benefit from documenting exposure, seeking medical evaluation, and requesting reasonable accommodations. Occupational health recognition of fragrance exposure as a legitimate hazard remains essential for policy change.

Fragrance Sensitivity and the Americans with Disabilities Act: Legal Standards and Case Law

Under the Americans with Disabilities Act of 1990 (ADA), employers with fifteen or more employees are required to provide reasonable accommodations to qualified individuals with disabilities unless doing so would impose undue hardship (Americans with Disabilities Act of 1990, 42 U.S.C. § 12101).

A disability is defined as a physical or mental impairment that substantially limits one or more major life activities. Major life activities include breathing, concentrating, neurological function, immune function, and working. The ADA Amendments Act of 2008 broadened the interpretation of "substantially limits" and clarified that the definition of disability should be construed in favor of broad coverage (ADA Amendments Act of 2008).

Fragrance sensitivity may qualify for protection when exposure to workplace chemicals substantially limits major life activities. Courts have recognized that environmental sensitivities, including chemical exposure, can meet ADA criteria when properly documented.

Key Legal Standards

To establish protection under the ADA, an employee must demonstrate:

1. A qualifying impairment
2. Substantial limitation of one or more major life activities
3. Ability to perform essential job functions with or without reasonable accommodation
4. If these elements are satisfied, the employer must engage in a good faith interactive process to determine an effective accommodation.

Relevant Case Law

McBride v. City of Detroit

In McBride v. City of Detroit, 2011 WL 6118563 (E.D. Mich. 2011), the court acknowledged that chemical sensitivity may qualify as a disability if it substantially limits major life activities. The ruling emphasized the need for individualized assessment rather than categorical exclusion.

Core v. Champaign County Board of County Commissioners

In Core v. Champaign County Board of County Commissioners, 2012 WL 3078814 (S.D. Ohio 2012), the court recognized that fragrance exposure triggering migraines and respiratory symptoms could constitute a disability under the ADA when supported by medical evidence demonstrating substantial limitation.

Brady v. United Refrigeration, Inc.

In Brady v. United Refrigeration, Inc., 2015 WL 3500125 (E.D. Pa. 2015), the court reaffirmed that employers must engage in the interactive process once aware of a disability and cannot summarily dismiss accommodation requests without evaluation.

ADA Amendments Act Impact

The ADA Amendments Act of 2008 significantly lowered the threshold for establishing disability status. Courts now focus less on whether the impairment qualifies and more on whether reasonable accommodation was provided (ADA Amendments Act of 2008).

Reasonable Accommodation in Fragrance Cases

Courts have identified the following as potentially reasonable accommodations depending on circumstances:

- Relocation of workstation
- Modification of workplace policies
- Installation of air filtration systems
- Remote work arrangements
- Implementation of limited fragrance free zones

Employer Obligations

Once an employer has notice of a disability, it must:

- Engage in an interactive process
- Evaluate proposed accommodations
- Provide effective accommodation unless undue hardship is proven

Failure to engage in this process can independently violate the ADA, even if the ultimate accommodation is disputed (Brady v. United Refrigeration, Inc., 2015).

Practical Legal Guidance

Employees seeking protection should:

- Obtain medical documentation clearly linking fragrance exposure to substantial limitation
- Submit a written ADA accommodation request
- Propose specific reasonable accommodations
- Document all employer responses

If accommodation is denied, employees may file a charge with the Equal Employment Opportunity Commission within 180 to 300 days depending on state law.

Conclusion

Fragrance sensitivity can qualify as a protected disability when it substantially limits breathing, neurological function, immune function, or the ability to work. Post 2008 ADA jurisprudence favors broad coverage and individualized analysis. Employers must engage in the interactive process and provide reasonable accommodation unless they can demonstrate undue hardship.

Occupational exposure to synthetic fragrance represents a significant and under-recognized workplace health risk. Exposure intensity varies by occupation, but prolonged daily contact substantially increases neurological, respiratory, hormonal, and immune stress. With reported health effects affecting up to one third of exposed workers in some settings, fragrance exposure can no longer be considered benign. Fragrance free workplace practices represent a practical, evidence based approach to protecting employee health, improving indoor air quality, and supporting inclusive work environments. Reducing occupational fragrance exposure is not optional comfort. It is a matter of public and occupational health.

Health Risks:
Killed by Fragrance

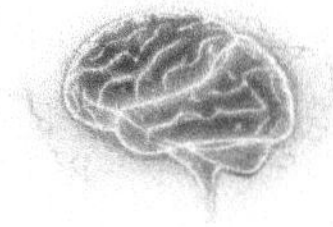
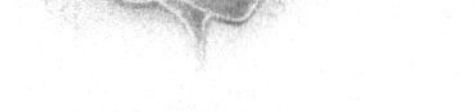

The Nervous System

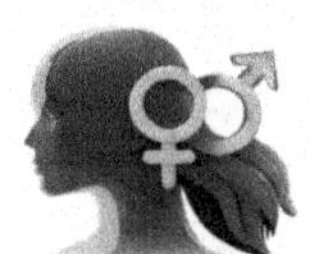

Hormonal Disruption

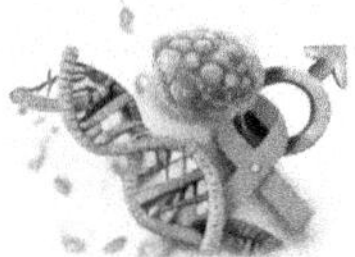

Cancer Risk

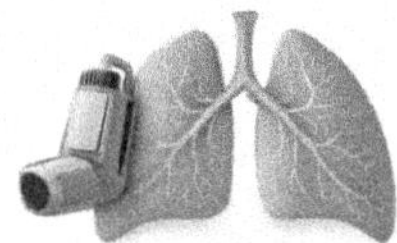

Asthma & COPD

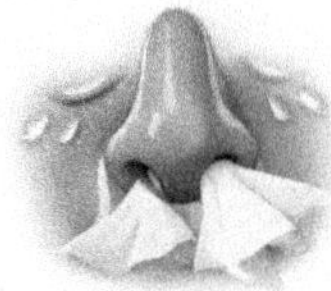
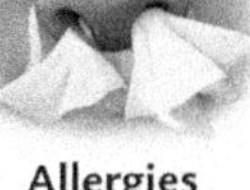

Allergies

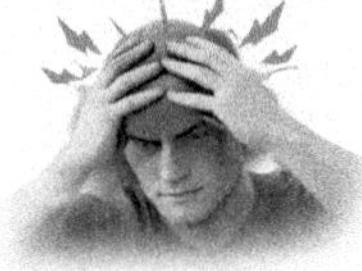

Migraines

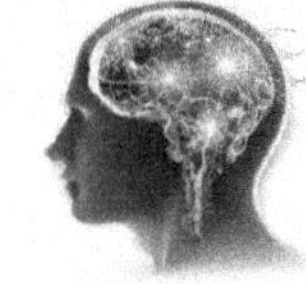

Neurological Disorders

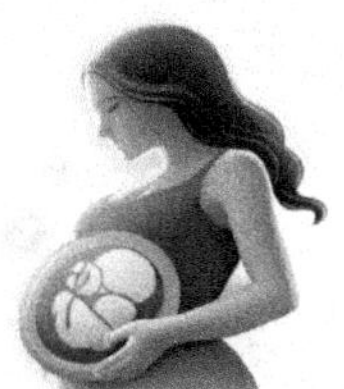

Fertility & Pregnancy

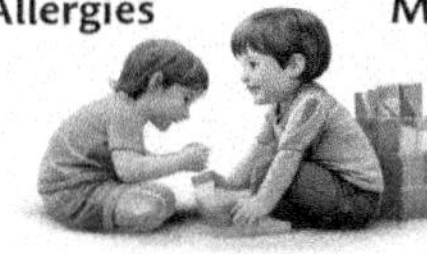

Children & Development

1. The Nervous System

1. The Nervous System

The nervous system is one of the most sensitive and directly affected targets of synthetic fragrance exposure. Unlike many organs that encounter chemicals only after metabolic processing, the nervous system is exposed through direct sensory and inhalation pathways. **Fragrance chemicals are intentionally designed to activate the olfactory and trigeminal nerve systems, and their neurological effects are supported by established physiological mechanisms and documented research.**

Direct Neural Exposure Through Smell

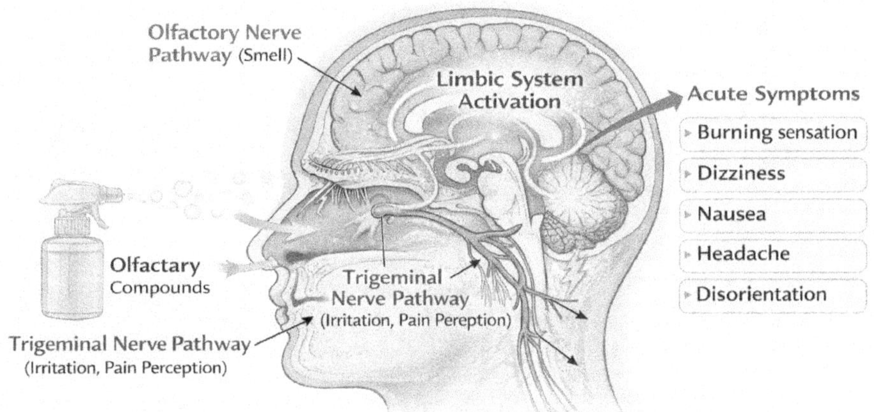

The trigeminal system mediates irritation, pain perception, and autonomic reflexes. Activation of these pathways explains acute symptoms such as burning sensations, dizziness, nausea, and disorientation reported after fragrance exposure.

The olfactory system provides a direct interface between the external environment and the brain. Olfactory receptor neurons project directly to the olfactory bulb, bypassing the blood brain barrier. This anatomical pathway allows airborne chemicals to access central nervous system structures without hepatic detoxification or systemic filtration (Doty, 2001). Fragrance compounds readily stimulate both olfactory and trigeminal nerve pathways. The trigeminal system mediates irritation, pain perception, and autonomic reflexes. Activation of these pathways explains acute symptoms such as burning sensations, dizziness, nausea, headache, and disorientation reported after fragrance exposure (Doty et al., 2004).

Limbic System Activation and Emotional Regulation

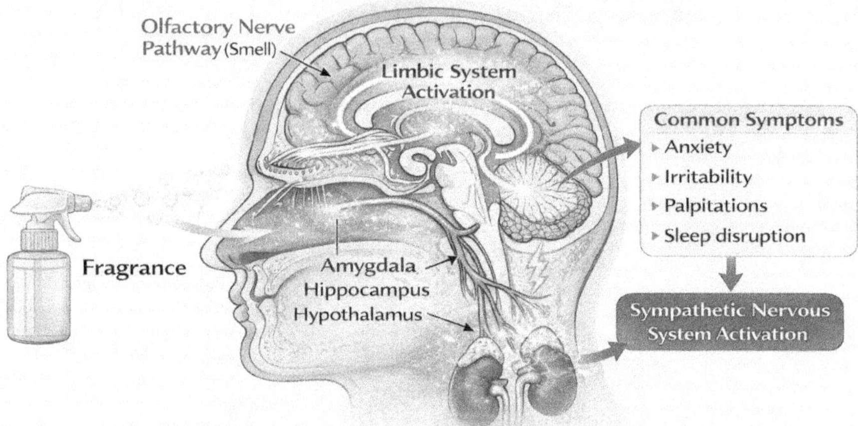

Clinical observations document increased sympathetic nervous system activation following fragrance exposure. Symptoms include anxiety, irritability, palpitations, sleep disruption, and

Neural signals from the olfactory bulb project directly to limbic structures, including the amygdala and hippocampus. These regions regulate emotion, memory, stress response, and autonomic balance. Neurophysiological studies demonstrate that odorant exposure rapidly alters limbic activity, influencing anxiety levels, mood, and stress hormone release (Herz, 2009). Clinical observations document increased sympathetic nervous system activation following fragrance exposure. Symptoms include anxiety, irritability, palpitations, sleep disruption, and heightened stress responses, particularly in vulnerable individuals (Anderson & Anderson, 1998).

Migraines and Headache Disorders

Fragrance is among the most commonly reported migraine triggers. Epidemiological studies indicate that a significant proportion of individuals with migraine experience attacks following exposure to scented products (Kelman, 2007). Mechanistic research supports involvement of trigeminovascular pathways, leading to neurogenic inflammation and sensitization of pain circuits. Repeated exposure may lower migraine thresholds over time, contributing to chronic migraine patterns and increased neurological sensitivity.

Neurotoxicity of Volatile Organic Compounds

Many fragrance ingredients are volatile organic compounds with known neuroactive properties. Human and animal studies demonstrate that inhalation exposure to VOCs can impair attention, memory, processing speed, and cognitive performance (Mendell, 2004). Population surveys consistently report brain fog, difficulty concentrating, and mental fatigue associated with fragrance exposure (Steinemann, 2018). Occupational studies further link chronic exposure to neurobehavioral impairment, reinforcing the impact of sustained low dose exposure in enclosed environments (Kilburn, 2000).

Autonomic Nervous System Dysregulation

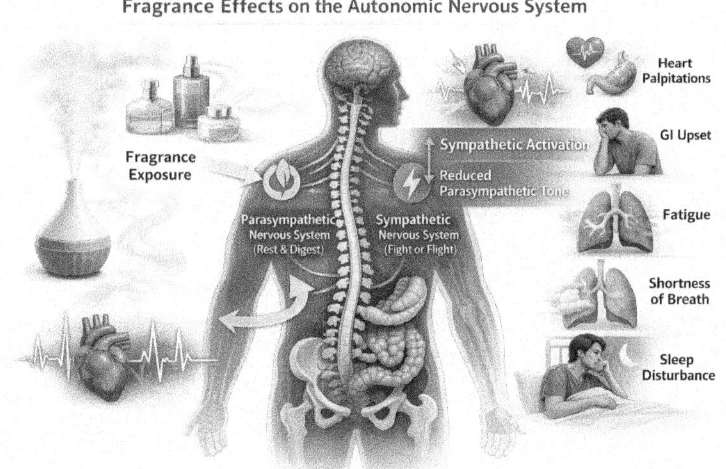

1. The Nervous System

The autonomic nervous system regulates involuntary physiological processes including heart rate, respiration, digestion, and stress response. Experimental studies demonstrate that fragrance exposure can shift autonomic balance toward sympathetic dominance with reduced parasympathetic tone (Dalton, 2003). This dysregulation contributes to symptoms such as palpitations, gastrointestinal discomfort, fatigue, shortness of breath, and sleep disturbance. Individuals with migraines, anxiety disorders, or chronic illness often exhibit heightened susceptibility.

Neuroinflammation and Sensitization

Repeated chemical exposure may lead to neuroinflammation and central sensitization. Research on chemical sensitivity syndromes demonstrates that repeated low level exposures can amplify neural responsiveness, resulting in exaggerated symptoms upon subsequent exposure (Bell et al., 2001). Neuroinflammatory processes involve glial activation, cytokine release, and altered neurotransmitter signaling. These mechanisms explain why symptoms often worsen over time rather than resolve with continued exposure.

Developmental Vulnerability

The developing nervous system is particularly susceptible to chemical insult. Prenatal and early childhood exposure to neuroactive chemicals has been associated with altered neurodevelopment, behavioral changes, and cognitive effects (Grandjean & Landrigan, 2014). Children inhale more air per body weight and have immature detoxification systems, increasing vulnerability.

Clinical and Occupational Evidence

Clinical case reports document improvement in neurological symptoms following fragrance avoidance, including reductions in headaches, improved cognition, decreased anxiety, and better sleep quality (Ziem & McTamney, 1997). Occupational studies demonstrate higher prevalence of headaches, dizziness, and cognitive complaints among workers in fragranced environments (Steinemann, 2018).

Conclusion

The neurological effects of synthetic fragrance exposure are not subjective, psychosomatic, or incidental. They represent predictable outcomes of chemical interaction with highly sensitive neural pathways. Fragrance chemicals are intentionally designed to stimulate sensory systems, yet repeated stimulation in enclosed environments produces neurological stress, autonomic imbalance, and neuroinflammatory responses. **Recognizing fragrance exposure as a neurological stressor reframes symptoms often dismissed as anxiety or stress as biologically grounded responses to chemical exposure**. This understanding is essential for accurate diagnosis, effective intervention, and prevention of chronic neurological dysfunction.

2. Hormonal Disruption

The endocrine system regulates nearly every critical function in the human body, including metabolism, growth, reproduction, stress response, immune balance, and neurological signaling. Hormones operate at extremely low concentrations, which makes the endocrine system uniquely sensitive to chemical interference. Synthetic fragrance exposure introduces compounds that are capable of disrupting hormonal signaling through multiple mechanisms, often at doses far below those traditionally considered toxic.

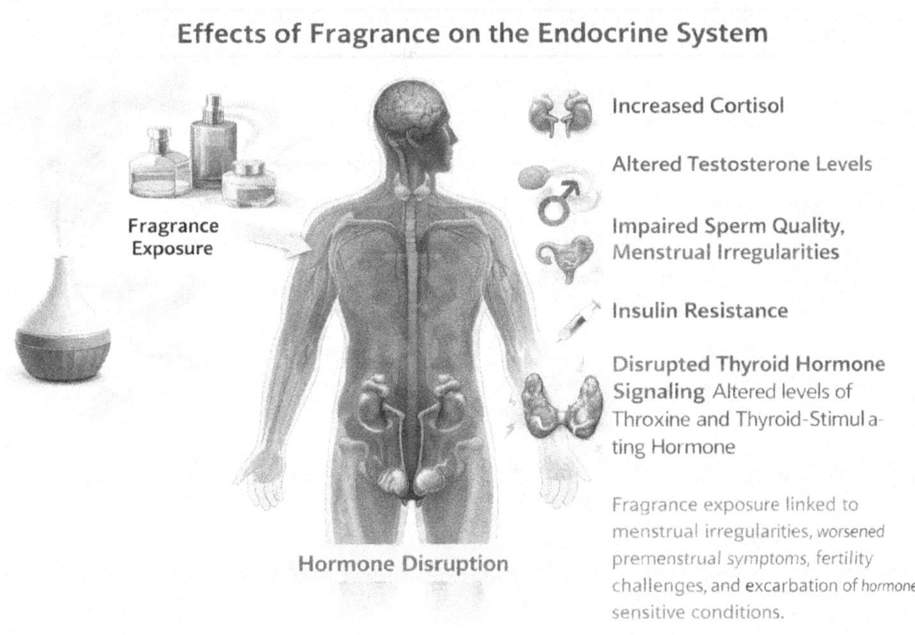

Endocrine Disrupting Chemicals in Fragrance

Many fragrance ingredients are classified as endocrine disrupting chemicals. These compounds interfere with hormone synthesis, transport, metabolism, receptor binding, or signaling pathways (Gore et al., 2015). Fragrance related endocrine disruptors include phthalates, synthetic musks, phenols, and certain aldehydes, many of which are undisclosed due to trade secret protections (Steinemann, 2016). Unlike acute toxins, endocrine disruptors exert effects through chronic low dose exposure. This exposure pattern aligns precisely with how fragranced products are used. Daily application, inhalation, and dermal contact create sustained hormonal interference over time.

Phthalates and Hormonal Interference

Phthalates are among the most extensively studied fragrance related endocrine disruptors. They are commonly used as fixatives to stabilize and prolong scent. Human biomonitoring studies consistently detect phthalate metabolites in urine, blood, and amniotic fluid, confirming widespread exposure (Meeker et al., 2009). Research demonstrates that phthalates exhibit estrogenic and antiandrogenic activity. Epidemiological studies link phthalate exposure to altered testosterone levels, impaired sperm quality, menstrual irregularities, insulin resistance, and disrupted thyroid hormone signaling (Meeker et al., 2009; Gore et al., 2015). Prenatal exposure is of particular concern. Studies associate maternal phthalate exposure with altered reproductive development and neurobehavioral outcomes in offspring, highlighting long term consequences of early hormonal disruption (Swan et al., 2015).

Thyroid Disruption

The thyroid gland plays a central role in metabolic regulation, energy production, and neurological development. Several fragrance related chemicals interfere with thyroid hormone synthesis, transport, and receptor binding. Phthalates and synthetic musks have been associated with altered levels of thyroxine and thyroid stimulating hormone in human studies (Boas et al., 2012). Disruption of thyroid signaling can manifest as fatigue, weight changes, cold intolerance, mood disturbance, and cognitive impairment. Because thyroid hormones interact with nearly every tissue, even modest disruption can produce widespread symptoms.

Estrogen and Progesterone Imbalance

Synthetic fragrance chemicals can alter estrogen and progesterone balance through receptor interaction and metabolic interference. Certain fragrance compounds demonstrate estrogen receptor agonist activity, while others inhibit hormone metabolism, leading to hormonal imbalance (Diamanti Kandarakis et al., 2009). Clinical observations link fragrance exposure to menstrual irregularities, worsened premenstrual symptoms, fertility challenges, and exacerbation of hormone sensitive conditions. Although causality is multifactorial, mechanistic and epidemiological data provide evidence of a biological basis for these observed effects.

Cortisol and Stress Hormone Dysregulation

The hypothalamic pituitary adrenal axis is highly responsive to chemical stressors. Fragrance exposure has been shown to activate stress pathways through sensory and neurological mechanisms, leading to increased cortisol release and autonomic imbalance (Herz, 2009). Chronic activation of stress hormones contributes to insulin resistance, immune suppression, sleep disruption, and mood disorders. When fragrance exposure is constant, the endocrine stress response may remain persistently activated, compounding metabolic and hormonal dysfunction.

Bioaccumulation and Long Term Exposure

Many fragrance chemicals are lipophilic and bioaccumulative. Synthetic musks have been detected in human adipose tissue, breast milk, and umbilical cord blood, indicating chronic exposure and potential transgenerational transfer (Reiner et al., 2007). Because hormones operate in feedback loops, accumulated endocrine disruptors may exert prolonged effects even after exposure reduction. This persistence complicates diagnosis and recovery.

Vulnerable Populations

Certain populations demonstrate heightened vulnerability to hormonal disruption. Fetuses, infants, children, and adolescents undergo critical periods of endocrine development. Exposure during these windows can produce lasting effects on growth, metabolism, and reproductive health (Gore et al., 2015). Individuals with existing endocrine disorders, including thyroid disease, polycystic ovary syndrome, diabetes, or adrenal dysfunction, may experience amplified effects from fragrance related endocrine disruption.

Clinical and Epidemiological Evidence

2. Hormonal Disruption

Population studies consistently associate fragrance related endocrine disruptors with hormonal abnormalities across multiple systems. While individual studies vary in design, the convergence of human biomonitoring, animal models, and mechanistic research supports a causal role for fragrance chemicals in endocrine dysfunction (Diamanti Kandarakis et al., 2009; Gore et al., 2015). Clinical case reports document symptom improvement following reduction or elimination of fragranced product exposure, further supporting the role of fragrance as a modifiable endocrine stressor.

Conclusion

Hormonal disruption from synthetic fragrance exposure represents a significant and underrecognized contributor to modern endocrine dysfunction. Fragrance chemicals interfere with hormone signaling at multiple levels, including receptor binding, hormone synthesis, metabolism, and feedback regulation. These effects occur at low doses, accumulate over time, and disproportionately affect vulnerable populations. Recognizing fragrance exposure as a potential endocrine disruptor reframes unexplained hormonal symptoms as biologically grounded responses to chemical interference rather than isolated dysfunction. Reducing fragrance exposure represents a meaningful and actionable step toward restoring hormonal balance and protecting long term endocrine health.

3. Cancer Risk

Cancer risk associated with synthetic fragrance exposure is best understood by examining how specific chemical mechanisms interact with different tissues. Fragrance related compounds influence cancer risk through endocrine disruption, genotoxicity, oxidative stress, immune modulation, and bioaccumulation. These mechanisms do not affect all tissues equally. Certain organs demonstrate heightened vulnerability based on hormone sensitivity, exposure route, and developmental timing.

Thyroid Cancer

The thyroid gland is particularly vulnerable to chemical disruption due to its reliance on precise hormonal signaling and iodine transport. Several fragrance related chemicals, including phthalates and synthetic musks, have been shown to interfere with thyroid hormone synthesis, transport, and receptor activity (Boas et al., 2012). Epidemiological studies link exposure to endocrine disrupting chemicals with altered thyroid hormone levels and increased thyroid disease prevalence. Thyroid disruption during critical windows of development is associated with long term thyroid dysfunction and increased cancer susceptibility. Because thyroid cancer risk is influenced by hormonal dysregulation and environmental exposures, chronic contact with fragrance related endocrine disrupting compounds warrants consideration as a potential risk factor supported by mechanistic evidence (Gore et al., 2015). Formaldehyde exposure further compounds risk. Formaldehyde and formaldehyde releasing compounds can be generated as secondary pollutants from fragrance terpene reactions indoors. Formaldehyde is a recognized human carcinogen with documented effects on endocrine and epithelial tissues (IARC, 2012).

Breast Cancer

Breast tissue is highly sensitive to estrogenic signaling. Fragrance related endocrine disruptors including phthalates, phenols, and synthetic musks demonstrate estrogen receptor activity and interference with hormone metabolism (Diamanti Kandarakis et al., 2009). Human biomonitoring studies consistently detect fragrance related compounds in breast tissue and breast milk, indicating direct exposure of mammary tissue (Reiner et al., 2007). Animal and mechanistic studies suggest that estrogenic chemicals may promote abnormal cell proliferation, reduce apoptosis, and increase susceptibility to malignant transformation. Early life exposure is particularly concerning. Developmental exposure to endocrine disruptors has been associated with altered mammary gland development and increased cancer susceptibility later in life (Gore et al., 2015).

Prostate Cancer

The prostate gland is regulated by androgen signaling, making it vulnerable to antiandrogenic endocrine disruptors. Phthalates used in fragrance fixation exhibit antiandrogenic effects and have been associated with altered testosterone levels and prostate development in experimental and epidemiological studies (Meeker et al., 2009). Chronic endocrine disruption may contribute to prostate tissue dysregulation, inflammation, and increased cancer susceptibility over time. While direct causation is difficult to establish, the biological mechanisms linking antiandrogenic exposure to prostate cancer risk are well supported.

Skin Cancer

The skin represents both a barrier and a primary exposure route for fragrance chemicals. Many fragranced personal care products are applied directly to the skin multiple times per day. Dermal absorption allows fragrance compounds to penetrate into deeper layers where they may induce oxidative stress and DNA damage. Phototoxic fragrance compounds, including certain synthetic musks and fragrance terpenes, can generate reactive oxygen species when exposed to ultraviolet radiation. This interaction increases oxidative stress in skin cells and may contribute to mutagenesis and carcinogenesis (Api et al., 2015). Repeated dermal exposure to fragrance related compounds, in conjunction with ultraviolet radiation, may contribute to mechanisms associated with increased skin cancer risk, particularly with prolonged use of fragranced cosmetics and sunscreens.

Hematologic Cancers

Certain fragrance related solvents and benzene derivatives raise concern for hematologic malignancies. Benzene is a well established human carcinogen linked to leukemia and bone marrow suppression. While fragrance related exposures are typically lower than occupational benzene exposure, chronic low dose inhalation in enclosed environments contributes to cumulative risk (Lan et al., 2004). Indoor air chemistry studies demonstrate that fragranced products contribute to volatile organic compound load, increasing the potential for systemic exposure through inhalation.

Hormone Sensitive Cancers Overall

Beyond individual cancer types, fragrance related endocrine disruption may increase overall risk for hormone sensitive cancers. Disruption of estrogen, androgen, thyroid, and cortisol signaling alters cell proliferation, immune surveillance, and apoptosis. These pathways are central to cancer initiation and progression (Diamanti Kandarakis et al., 2009). Because endocrine disruptors often exhibit nonmonotonic dose responses, low dose chronic exposure may produce effects not predicted by traditional toxicology models.

Occupational and Early Life Exposure

Cancer risk is influenced by duration and timing of exposure. Occupational settings such as healthcare, salons, cleaning services, and manufacturing environments involve prolonged fragrance exposure in enclosed spaces. Early life exposure during fetal development and childhood further increases vulnerability due to rapid cell division and immature detoxification systems (Grandjean & Landrigan, 2014).

Carcinogenic Chemicals Hidden in Fragrance Formulations

When consumers see the word "fragrance" or "perfume" on a label, they are not seeing a single ingredient. They are seeing a legal placeholder that can represent dozens or even hundreds of undisclosed chemicals. While it is difficult to find studies that test "fragrance" as a single exposure and directly conclude "fragrance causes cancer," many chemicals commonly used in fragranced products have been independently evaluated by the International Agency for Research on Cancer (IARC), the World Health Organization (WHO), the U.S. Environmental Protection Agency (EPA), and other regulatory bodies and classified as carcinogenic or potentially carcinogenic to humans. These substances are frequently found in perfumes, body sprays, lotions, sunscreens, air fresheners, candles, detergents, and other personal care products.

Common Fragrance-Related Chemicals with Carcinogenic Classifications

Below is a summary of well-documented ingredients that have been classified as carcinogenic or possibly carcinogenic based on human, animal, or mechanistic data.

Potentially Carcinogenic Ingredients Hidden in Fragrance			
Ingredient	**Common Use in Fragrance & Personal Care**	**Classification**	**Evidence Level**
Benzene	Contaminant in aerosols, sunscreens, sprays	Group 1 Carcinogen (IARC)	High
Formaldehyde	Preservative, fragrance stabilizer	Group 1 Carcinogen (IARC)	High
1,4-Dioxane	Contaminant in ethoxylated surfactants	Probable Human Carcinogen	High
Ethylene Oxide	Sterilization, residual contamination	Group 1 Carcinogen	High
Styrene	Fragrance component, plastics	Group 2A (Probable)	Medium–High
Acetaldehyde	Fragrance component	Group 2B (Possible)	Medium
BHA (Butylated Hydroxyanisole)	Fragrance preservative	Group 2B	Medium
Titanium Dioxide (inhaled, aerosol form)	Sunscreen sprays	Group 2B	Medium
Carbon Black (inhaled)	Pigment in cosmetics	Group 2B	Medium
Diethyl Phthalate (DEP)	Fragrance fixative	Group 2B	Medium
Nitrosamines (NDMA, NDEA)	Endocrine-disrupting; tumor-promoting potential	Group 2B	Medium

The "classification" column in this table refers to how major scientific and regulatory bodies categorize a substance based on its cancer-causing potential in humans. Classifications such as Group 1, Group 2A, and Group 2B come from evaluations conducted by international health authorities and reflect the strength of scientific agreement that a substance can cause cancer. Group 1 indicates there is sufficient evidence in humans that the substance is carcinogenic. Group 2A, classified as "probably carcinogenic," means there is strong evidence from animal studies and supportive mechanistic data, with limited but concerning human evidence. Group 2B, labeled "possibly carcinogenic," indicates more limited human evidence but credible concern based on experimental or mechanistic findings.

The "evidence level" column summarizes how strong and consistent the overall body of research is regarding cancer risk. A "High" evidence level means multiple well-conducted studies, including human epidemiological data, support carcinogenic potential. "Medium–High" reflects strong animal or mechanistic data with growing human concern. "Medium" indicates emerging or limited human evidence combined with biological plausibility. Together, these two columns help the reader distinguish between confirmed human carcinogens and chemicals with significant but varying degrees of documented cancer risk.

High-Probability Carcinogens (Group 1 – Carcinogenic to Humans)

Benzene

Benzene exposure is strongly linked to leukemia and other blood cancers (IARC, 2018). Although not intentionally added to cosmetic formulations, benzene has been detected as a contaminant in aerosol sunscreens, body sprays, deodorant sprays, dry shampoo, and certain spray hand sanitizers. Because these products are applied directly to the skin or sprayed into the air, inhalation becomes a primary route of exposure. Chronic low-level inhalation exposure is particularly concerning due to benzene's well-established hematologic toxicity (Smith, 2010).

Formaldehyde

Formaldehyde is classified as carcinogenic to humans and is associated with nasopharyngeal cancer and leukemia (IARC, 2012). In consumer products, formaldehyde may be present directly in some hair smoothing treatments, nail products, and disinfectants, or it may be slowly released from formaldehyde-releasing preservatives commonly used in shampoos, body washes, lotions, cosmetics, and fragranced cleaning agents. Inhalation exposure in enclosed indoor environments is the primary concern.

Ethylene Oxide

Ethylene oxide is a known human carcinogen linked to breast cancer and lymphoid cancers (Steenland et al., 2004). While not intentionally used as a fragrance ingredient, it is commonly used to sterilize medical equipment, cosmetics, and certain raw materials used in personal care manufacturing. Residual contamination can remain in products such as wipes, medical dressings, and some cosmetic ingredients that undergo ethoxylation processing. Chronic trace exposure is a concern due to its DNA-reactive properties.

Medium-Probability Carcinogens (Group 2A and 2B)

Styrene

Styrene has been classified as probably carcinogenic to humans based on occupational exposure studies linking it to hematologic malignancies (IARC, 2019). In consumer settings, styrene may be present in fragranced plastics, cosmetic packaging, air fresheners, scented candles, and certain synthetic fragrance compounds. Off-gassing from scented plastic materials can contribute to indoor air exposure.

Titanium Dioxide (Aerosolized Form)

While considered relatively stable in solid topical form, inhaled titanium dioxide particles, particularly in spray sunscreens, cosmetic powders, and aerosol personal care products, are classified as possibly carcinogenic (IARC, 2010). Risk is primarily associated with airborne inhalation rather than skin contact.

Carbon Black (Inhaled)

Carbon black, when inhaled chronically, has demonstrated carcinogenic potential in animal models (IARC, 2010). It is commonly used as a pigment in mascara, eyeliner, cosmetics, hair dyes, and certain fragranced sprays. In powder or aerosolized form, inhalation exposure becomes relevant.

Phthalates

Phthalates such as diethyl phthalate are widely used as fragrance stabilizers and fixatives to help scents last longer. They are commonly found in perfumes, colognes, body lotions, deodorants, hair sprays, and air fresheners. While not universally classified as direct carcinogens, phthalates are well-documented endocrine disruptors. Hormonal disruption is increasingly recognized as a contributing pathway in hormone-sensitive cancers such as breast and prostate cancer (Diamanti-Kandarakis et al., 2009).

Why "Fragrance" Itself Is Rarely Studied as a Single Variable

One of the challenges in researching cancer risk related to fragrance exposure is regulatory labeling. "Fragrance" is legally protected as a trade secret. Researchers cannot easily isolate or standardize exposure across products because formulations vary widely and are not fully disclosed. However, toxicology does not operate in a vacuum. If a mixture contains substances that are independently classified as carcinogenic, then the mixture inherits that risk potential depending on dose, frequency, route of exposure, and cumulative burden. Inhalation is particularly significant. The respiratory epithelium provides direct access to systemic circulation. Repeated daily exposure through perfumes, scented lotions, candles, and aerosol sunscreens creates chronic low-dose exposure scenarios that have not been thoroughly evaluated in long-term cumulative models.

The Cumulative Exposure Problem

Most individuals do not use just one fragranced product. A typical day may include:

- Scented body wash
- Shampoo and conditioner
- Deodorant
- Perfume or cologne
- Laundry detergent residue
- Fabric softener
- Sunscreen
- Indoor air fresheners

Each application may appear small in isolation. However, cumulative exposure across years raises legitimate mechanistic concern, particularly when known carcinogens or probable carcinogens are present.

Summary of Evidence

3. Cancer Risk

It is difficult to locate a single study that states, "Fragrance increases cancer risk," because fragrance is not one chemical. It is a complex and undisclosed mixture.

However:

- Multiple chemicals commonly found in fragranced personal care and sunscreen products are classified by the WHO and IARC as carcinogenic or possibly carcinogenic.
- Some are confirmed human carcinogens.
- Others are endocrine disruptors that may promote hormone-sensitive tumor development.
- Aerosolized products increase inhalation exposure, a known high-risk route for certain carcinogens.

Therefore, while direct mixture-level epidemiologic data may be limited, the presence of independently classified carcinogenic substances in frequently used consumer products raises legitimate concern about increased cancer risk under chronic exposure conditions.

Precaution is not alarmism. It is informed risk assessment.

4. Asthma and COPD

The respiratory system is a primary target of synthetic fragrance exposure. Because fragranced chemicals are designed to volatilize and disperse into indoor air, inhalation represents one of the most direct and biologically impactful exposure routes. For individuals with asthma, chronic obstructive pulmonary disease, or underlying airway sensitivity, fragrance exposure can provoke acute symptoms, worsen disease control, and accelerate long term respiratory decline.

Respiratory Sensitivity to Fragrance Chemicals

The airways are lined with delicate epithelial tissue that serves as both a barrier and a sensory interface. Fragrance chemicals readily interact with this tissue, activating irritant receptors and inflammatory pathways. Volatile organic compounds commonly emitted from fragranced products stimulate the trigeminal nerve and airway sensory nerves, leading to bronchoconstriction, cough, and airway irritation (Dalton, 2003). Unlike particulate pollutants that may settle or be filtered, fragrance chemicals remain airborne and are easily inhaled deep into the lungs, particularly in enclosed indoor environments.

Asthma Exacerbation

Asthma is characterized by airway hyperresponsiveness, inflammation, and reversible airflow obstruction. Fragrance exposure is a well documented trigger for asthma symptoms and attacks. Epidemiological studies consistently report increased wheezing, shortness of breath, chest tightness, and coughing following exposure to fragranced consumer products (Caress & Steinemann, 2009). Controlled exposure studies demonstrate that inhalation of fragrance related volatile organic compounds can induce bronchoconstriction and increase airway resistance even in individuals with mild or well controlled asthma. Repeated exposure lowers the threshold for future attacks, contributing to poor asthma control over time (Anderson & Anderson, 1998).

Chronic Obstructive Pulmonary Disease (COPD)

Chronic obstructive pulmonary disease is characterized by persistent airflow limitation, chronic inflammation, and progressive lung damage. Individuals with COPD exhibit heightened sensitivity to inhaled irritants due to compromised airway defenses and reduced pulmonary reserve. Fragrance exposure can provoke acute symptom exacerbations in COPD, including increased dyspnea, cough, and mucus production. Inflammatory responses triggered by volatile organic compounds may further damage airway epithelium and contribute to disease progression (Mølhave et al., 2000). Because COPD symptoms may worsen gradually, fragrance related contributions are often overlooked, yet avoidance studies demonstrate symptom improvement when exposure is reduced.

Airway Inflammation and Immune Activation

Fragrance chemicals can activate inflammatory pathways within the respiratory tract. In vitro and human exposure studies demonstrate increased release of inflammatory mediators, oxidative stress markers, and epithelial irritation following VOC inhalation (Mendell, 2004). Chronic airway inflammation contributes to remodeling of bronchial tissue, increased mucus production, and reduced lung function. These changes are central to both asthma and COPD pathology.

Occupational Exposure and Respiratory Risk

Occupational settings present heightened risk due to sustained exposure in enclosed spaces. Healthcare workers, cleaners, educators, salon professionals, and service industry employees are frequently exposed to fragranced products throughout the workday. Studies report higher prevalence of asthma symptoms, respiratory irritation, and work related breathing difficulties in these populations. Fragrance exposure is increasingly recognized as an occupational asthma trigger, yet remains inadequately addressed in workplace health policies (Steinemann, 2018).

Children and Early Life Exposure

Children are particularly vulnerable to fragrance related respiratory effects. They inhale more air per body weight than adults and have developing respiratory and immune systems. Exposure to fragranced products in homes, schools, and childcare settings has been associated with increased wheezing, asthma symptoms, and respiratory irritation (Caress & Steinemann, 2009).

Early life exposure during critical periods of lung development may increase long term susceptibility to chronic respiratory disease.

Misclassification and Underrecognition

Respiratory symptoms triggered by fragrance exposure are frequently mistaken for allergic reactions, anxiety, or nonspecific irritation. This misclassification delays proper identification of environmental triggers and results in continued exposure, allowing symptoms to persist or worsen. Clinical studies demonstrate that avoidance of fragranced products results in symptom reduction and improved respiratory function in susceptible individuals, supporting a causal relationship rather than coincidence (Ziem & McTamney, 1997).

Interaction With Other Air Pollutants

Fragrance chemicals do not act in isolation. Indoor air chemistry studies show that fragrance compounds react with ozone and other indoor pollutants to form secondary irritants such as formaldehyde and ultrafine particles. These secondary pollutants further aggravate airway inflammation and respiratory symptoms (Weschler & Shields, 1997). This interaction amplifies respiratory risk even when individual fragrance ingredients are present at low concentrations.

Conclusion

The respiratory system represents one of the most immediate and vulnerable targets of synthetic fragrance exposure. Because fragranced chemicals are intentionally engineered to volatilize and remain airborne, inhalation provides a direct route to the airway epithelium, sensory nerves, and lower respiratory tract. Mechanistic research, controlled exposure studies, epidemiological data, and occupational findings collectively demonstrate that fragrance related volatile organic compounds can provoke airway irritation, bronchoconstriction, inflammation, and symptom exacerbation, particularly in susceptible individuals.

For patients with asthma or chronic obstructive pulmonary disease, fragrance exposure is not a benign nuisance. It is a clinically relevant trigger capable of worsening symptom control, increasing airway hyperresponsiveness, and potentially contributing to long term disease progression. Even in individuals without diagnosed respiratory disease, repeated exposure may promote airway inflammation and heightened sensitivity over time.

Children, workers in high exposure occupations, and individuals with preexisting airway vulnerability face disproportionate risk. Additionally, the interaction of fragrance chemicals with ozone and other indoor pollutants generates secondary irritants that amplify respiratory burden beyond the original exposure. The cumulative evidence supports a precautionary and preventive approach. Recognition of fragrance exposure as a modifiable respiratory risk factor shifts the focus from symptom suppression to environmental intervention. Reducing or eliminating exposure to fragranced products, particularly in enclosed indoor environments and for individuals at elevated risk, represents a practical and preventive approach to safeguarding respiratory health.

5. Allergies

The immune system is designed to identify and neutralize harmful threats while maintaining tolerance to harmless substances. Synthetic fragrance exposure disrupts this balance by introducing complex chemical mixtures that can irritate immune tissues, activate inflammatory pathways, and promote allergic sensitization. Over time, repeated exposure may contribute to both classic allergic responses and broader immune dysregulation.

Fragrance as an Immune Trigger

Fragrance chemicals interact directly with immune cells located in the skin, respiratory tract, and mucosal surfaces. Many fragrance ingredients function as haptens, small molecules that bind to proteins and form antigenic complexes capable of triggering immune recognition. This process can initiate allergic sensitization even in individuals with no prior allergy history (Kimber et al., 2011). Once sensitization occurs, subsequent exposure may provoke exaggerated immune responses, leading to symptoms that intensify over time rather than resolve.

Allergic Contact Dermatitis

Allergic contact dermatitis is one of the most well documented immune reactions to fragrance exposure. Fragrance mixtures are among the leading causes of contact allergy worldwide. Patch testing studies consistently identify fragrance components as frequent sensitizers in patients with eczema and chronic skin inflammation (Johansen et al., 2011). Dermal exposure allows fragrance chemicals to penetrate the skin barrier and activate antigen presenting cells, leading to T cell mediated immune responses. Clinically, this manifests as redness, itching, swelling, rash, and chronic skin irritation. Repeated exposure increases sensitization risk, particularly when fragranced products are applied to compromised skin or used daily over extended periods.

Respiratory Allergic Responses

Fragrance exposure can provoke allergic and pseudoallergic reactions in the respiratory tract. Inhalation of volatile fragrance chemicals stimulates immune cells in airway mucosa, contributing to inflammation, mucus production, and airway hyperreactivity. Individuals with allergic rhinitis or asthma frequently report worsening symptoms following fragrance exposure, including nasal congestion, sneezing, throat irritation, and coughing. Epidemiological studies demonstrate strong associations between fragranced product exposure and upper respiratory symptoms in sensitized populations (Caress & Steinemann, 2009). Unlike classical pollen allergies, fragrance related respiratory reactions may occur year round due to continuous indoor exposure.

Mast Cell Activation and Histamine Release

Fragrance chemicals may directly activate mast cells, leading to histamine release independent of IgE mediated allergy. This mechanism explains why some individuals experience allergic type symptoms without positive allergy testing. Histamine release contributes to itching, flushing, headaches, nasal congestion, and gastrointestinal discomfort. Repeated mast cell activation may lower response thresholds and promote chronic symptom patterns.

Immune System Sensitization and Escalation

Repeated low dose chemical exposure can drive immune sensitization. Animal and human studies indicate that chronic exposure to irritant chemicals increases immune responsiveness and lowers tolerance thresholds, resulting in amplified reactions to subsequent exposure (Bell et al., 2001). This sensitization process explains why individuals often report increasing symptom severity over time, expanding triggers, and reduced tolerance to fragranced environments.

Multiple Chemical Sensitivity and Immune Dysregulation

Multiple chemical sensitivity is characterized by multisystem symptoms triggered by low level chemical exposure. While diagnostic criteria remain debated, immune dysregulation is increasingly recognized as a contributing factor. Studies demonstrate altered cytokine profiles, inflammatory markers, and immune activation in individuals with chemical sensitivity syndromes. Fragrance exposure is one of the most commonly reported triggers in this population (Bell et al., 2001).

Vulnerable Populations

Children, individuals with atopic disease, and those with compromised immune systems are particularly vulnerable. Early life exposure during immune system development may influence allergic disease risk later in life. Occupational exposure further increases risk. Healthcare workers, educators, cleaners, and service workers experience repeated fragrance exposure that may contribute to chronic immune activation and allergic disease prevalence.

Diagnostic Challenges

Fragrance related allergic reactions are often underdiagnosed due to incomplete ingredient disclosure and nonspecific symptom presentation. Standard allergy testing may not capture fragrance mixture sensitivity, leading to misdiagnosis or dismissal of symptoms.Clinical improvement following fragrance avoidance provides strong evidence of causality, yet this approach is rarely emphasized in conventional allergy management.

Conclusion

Synthetic fragrance exposure represents a significant and underrecognized contributor to allergic disease and immune dysfunction. Through hapten formation, mast cell activation, and chronic immune sensitization, fragrance chemicals disrupt immune tolerance and promote inflammatory responses. Recognizing fragrance as an immune trigger reframes allergic symptoms as predictable biological reactions rather than unexplained sensitivity. Reducing fragrance exposure offers a practical and effective strategy for restoring immune balance, decreasing allergic burden, and protecting long term immune health.

6. Migraines

Migraines are complex neurological disorders characterized by recurrent, often debilitating headaches accompanied by sensory, gastrointestinal, and cognitive symptoms. While genetics play a role, environmental triggers are central to migraine initiation and progression. Among these triggers, synthetic fragrance exposure is one of the most frequently reported and consistently documented.

Fragrance as a Migraine Trigger

Population studies consistently identify fragrance and strong odors as leading migraine triggers. Surveys of individuals with migraine show that a substantial percentage report headache onset shortly after exposure to perfumes, air fresheners, cleaning products, and scented personal care items (Kelman, 2007). Unlike dietary or hormonal triggers that may act internally, fragrance exposure initiates migraine through direct sensory and neurological pathways. This makes fragrance one of the most immediate and unavoidable migraine triggers in daily life.

Trigeminal Nerve Activation

The trigeminal nerve plays a central role in migraine pathophysiology. It innervates facial structures, nasal passages, and meningeal blood vessels. Volatile fragrance chemicals activate trigeminal nerve endings in the nasal mucosa, triggering pain signaling pathways associated with migraine onset (Doty et al., 2004). Trigeminal activation leads to the release of neuropeptides such as calcitonin gene related peptide, substance P, and neurokinin A. These mediators promote vasodilation, neurogenic inflammation, and pain sensitization, all hallmark features of migraine attacks.

Sensory Processing and Central Sensitization

Individuals with migraine exhibit heightened sensory sensitivity, including increased responsiveness to light, sound, and smell. Functional imaging studies demonstrate altered sensory processing in migraine brains, making them particularly reactive to odor stimuli (Burstein et al., 2015). Repeated fragrance exposure may contribute to central sensitization, a process in which the nervous system becomes increasingly responsive to stimuli. Central sensitization lowers migraine thresholds and increases attack frequency and severity over time.

Limbic System and Emotional Modulation

Olfactory input directly influences limbic structures involved in emotion and stress regulation. Exposure to synthetic fragrances can alter limbic activity, increasing anxiety, irritability, and stress hormone release. These changes further prime migraine pathways by amplifying autonomic imbalance and cortical excitability (Herz, 2009). Stress induced by fragrance exposure may therefore act as both a direct trigger and an amplifier of migraine susceptibility.

Neurotoxicity and Cognitive Symptoms

Many migraine sufferers report cognitive symptoms such as brain fog, slowed thinking, and difficulty concentrating during and after attacks. Volatile organic compounds commonly found in fragrances have demonstrated neurotoxic effects that impair attention, memory, and cognitive performance in both experimental and occupational studies (Mendell, 2004). These neurotoxic effects may prolong postdrome symptoms and contribute to cumulative neurological burden in individuals with frequent migraine exposure.

Migraine Chronification

Chronic migraine develops when episodic attacks increase in frequency and become persistent. Environmental triggers play a significant role in this transition. Repeated exposure to fragrance chemicals may promote migraine chronification by sustaining neuroinflammation and sensory sensitization. Clinical observations indicate that migraine frequency and severity often improve following fragrance avoidance, supporting the role of fragrance as a modifiable trigger rather than an unavoidable condition (Ziem & McTamney, 1997).

Occupational and Public Exposure

Fragrance exposure is particularly problematic in workplaces, healthcare settings, schools, and public spaces where individuals cannot control environmental scents. Studies report that migraine sufferers frequently avoid public spaces or miss work due to fragrance induced headaches, contributing to reduced quality of life and productivity (Steinemann, 2018). This involuntary exposure underscores the need for greater recognition of fragrance as a neurological trigger rather than a personal preference issue.

Diagnostic Challenges

Migraine triggers are often identified through patient self report rather than objective testing. Because fragrance exposure is normalized, it may not be recognized as a trigger until patients intentionally reduce exposure and observe symptom improvement. Healthcare providers may underestimate the impact of fragrance due to limited training in environmental medicine, leading to missed opportunities for nonpharmacologic intervention.

Conclusion

Synthetic fragrance exposure represents a powerful and underrecognized trigger for migraines. Through activation of trigeminal nerve pathways, limbic system modulation, neuroinflammation, and central sensitization, fragrance chemicals can initiate and perpetuate migraine attacks. Recognizing fragrance as a neurological trigger reframes migraine management beyond medication alone. Reducing fragrance exposure offers a practical, low risk strategy to decrease migraine frequency, severity, and chronification. For many individuals, environmental control represents a critical step toward restoring neurological stability and improving quality of life.

7. Neurological Disorders

Neurological disorders are among the most serious and life altering consequences of environmental chemical exposure. The brain and nervous system are uniquely vulnerable due to their high lipid content, intense metabolic demand, and limited capacity for regeneration. Synthetic fragrance exposure introduces neuroactive chemicals that can cross biological barriers, induce neuroinflammation, disrupt neurotransmission, and accelerate neurodegenerative processes. While genetics influence susceptibility, environmental exposures play a decisive role in the onset and progression of many neurological diseases. Increasing scientific evidence links chronic exposure to volatile organic compounds and endocrine disrupting chemicals commonly found in fragranced products with heightened risk of neurodegeneration.

Shared Mechanisms of Neurodegeneration

Neurodegenerative diseases share common pathological mechanisms, including oxidative stress, mitochondrial dysfunction, protein misfolding, impaired detoxification, and chronic neuroinflammation. Environmental neurotoxins accelerate these processes by overwhelming antioxidant defenses and activating microglia, the immune cells of the central nervous system (Grandjean & Landrigan, 2014). Fragrance related chemicals are of particular concern because they are inhaled and absorbed through the skin, allowing repeated access to neural tissue over long periods of time.

Alzheimer's Disease and Dementia

Alzheimer's disease is the most common cause of dementia and is characterized by progressive memory loss, cognitive decline, and behavioral changes. Pathological hallmarks include beta amyloid plaque accumulation, tau protein dysfunction, synaptic loss, oxidative stress, and chronic neuroinflammation. Exposure to volatile organic compounds has been associated with impaired cognitive performance, reduced memory function, and increased markers of neuroinflammation in both experimental and population based studies (Kilburn, 2000; Calderón Garcidueñas et al., 2016). Long term exposure to indoor air pollutants, including fragranced volatile compounds, has been linked to accelerated cognitive decline in older adults (Power et al., 2016). Fragrance chemicals that bioaccumulate in lipid rich brain tissue may contribute to amyloidogenic processes by disrupting membrane integrity, increasing oxidative stress, and impairing cellular clearance mechanisms. Because Alzheimer's disease develops over decades, chronic low-dose exposure represents a contributing factor rather than an acute cause.

Parkinson's Disease

Parkinson's disease is a progressive neurodegenerative disorder characterized by the loss of dopaminergic neurons in the substantia nigra. Core features include tremor, rigidity, bradykinesia, postural instability, and later cognitive impairment. Environmental exposure to neurotoxic chemicals is a well established risk factor for Parkinson's disease. Studies consistently associate solvent and volatile organic compound exposure with increased Parkinson's disease incidence (Pezzoli & Cereda, 2013). Many fragrance related chemicals share structural and functional similarities with known neurotoxic solvents and demonstrate mitochondrial toxicity and oxidative stress induction in experimental models. Inhalation exposure is especially relevant. The olfactory pathway provides a direct route from the nasal cavity to the brain, bypassing the blood brain barrier. Early olfactory dysfunction is a recognized prodromal symptom of Parkinson's disease, supporting the hypothesis that inhaled neurotoxins contribute to disease initiation.

Amyotrophic Lateral Sclerosis

Amyotrophic lateral sclerosis is a progressive neurodegenerative disease affecting upper and lower motor neurons. While relatively rare, ALS has strong associations with environmental exposure, oxidative stress, and mitochondrial dysfunction. Occupational and environmental studies link chronic exposure to solvents and volatile chemicals with increased ALS risk. These exposures may promote glutamate excitotoxicity, oxidative injury, and impaired neuronal repair mechanisms (Gallo et al., 2016).

Neuroinflammatory Disorders and Sensitization

Chronic neuroinflammation is a unifying feature of many neurological diseases. Fragrance related chemicals activate inflammatory signaling within the brain by stimulating microglia and altering cytokine balance. This inflammatory state increases neuronal vulnerability and accelerates disease progression. Individuals with neurological sensitivity often report symptom exacerbation following fragrance exposure, including fatigue, headaches, cognitive dysfunction, sensory overload, and autonomic instability. These responses reflect neuroimmune interactions rather than psychological intolerance (Bell et al., 2001).

Cognitive Impairment and Brain Fog

Beyond diagnosed neurodegenerative disease, fragrance exposure is associated with reversible but clinically meaningful cognitive symptoms. Controlled exposure studies demonstrate impairments in attention, memory, processing speed, and executive function following volatile organic compound exposure at levels commonly found indoors (Mendell, 2004). Repeated exposure may reduce cognitive reserve over time, increasing vulnerability to age related cognitive decline and neurodegenerative disease.

Developmental and Lifelong Vulnerability

Neurological vulnerability spans the entire lifespan. Prenatal and early childhood exposure to neurotoxic chemicals has been linked to altered brain development, behavioral disorders, and reduced cognitive resilience later in life (Grandjean & Landrigan, 2014). Because fragrance exposure is widespread and often continuous, it contributes to cumulative neurotoxic burden beginning early in life and extending into older adulthood.

Conclusion

Neurological disorders, including Alzheimer's disease and Parkinson's disease, represent a critical frontier in understanding the long term consequences of synthetic fragrance exposure. Through oxidative stress, mitochondrial dysfunction, neuroinflammation, and direct neural access via inhalation pathways, fragrance related chemicals may contribute to cognitive decline and neurodegenerative disease risk. Recognizing fragrance as a modifiable neurotoxic stressor provides a powerful opportunity for prevention. Reducing fragrance exposure across the lifespan may help lower cumulative neurological burden, protect cognitive function, and support long term brain health.

8. Children and Neurodevelopment

The developing brain is uniquely sensitive to environmental exposure. From early pregnancy through adolescence, neurodevelopment depends on precisely timed biological processes that guide cell proliferation, migration, synapse formation, myelination, and neural pruning. Disruption during these critical windows can result in lasting structural and functional changes. Synthetic fragrance exposure introduces neuroactive and endocrine disrupting chemicals during these vulnerable periods, raising serious concerns for long term cognitive, behavioral, and neurological health.

Critical Windows of Brain Development

Neurodevelopment begins early in fetal life and continues through adolescence. During pregnancy, the fetal brain undergoes rapid cell division and differentiation, guided by hormonal and molecular signaling. After birth, neural circuits are refined through sensory input and environmental interaction. Environmental chemicals that interfere with these processes can alter brain architecture permanently. Because developmental systems lack redundancy, even subtle disruption during critical periods may have disproportionate effects (Grandjean & Landrigan, 2014).

Prenatal Exposure and the Placenta

Many fragrance related chemicals are lipophilic and readily cross the placenta. Human biomonitoring studies have detected phthalates, synthetic musks, and other fragrance associated compounds in amniotic fluid, umbilical cord blood, and fetal tissue, confirming direct prenatal exposure (Swan et al., 2015). Prenatal exposure to endocrine disrupting chemicals has been associated with altered brain development, behavioral changes, and impaired cognitive outcomes. Hormones such as thyroid hormone, estrogen, and cortisol play central roles in neurodevelopment. Disruption of these systems during gestation can impair neuronal migration, synapse formation, and myelination (Boas et al., 2012).

Endocrine Disruption and Brain Development

Thyroid hormones are essential for fetal and early childhood brain development. Even mild disruption of thyroid signaling during pregnancy has been linked to lower intelligence quotient, attention deficits, and motor delay in children (Boas et al., 2012). Fragrance related endocrine disruptors including phthalates interfere with thyroid hormone synthesis, transport, and receptor activity. Because fragrance exposure is chronic and often daily, cumulative endocrine interference during development is a significant concern.

Early Childhood Exposure and Sensory Overload

Infants and young children experience higher relative exposure to airborne chemicals because they breathe more air per body weight than adults. They also spend more time close to floors and surfaces where fragrance chemicals accumulate. Exposure during early childhood has been associated with increased irritability, sleep disturbance, attention problems, and sensory sensitivity. These effects are consistent with neurobehavioral findings observed in children exposed to volatile organic compounds in indoor environments (Mendell, 2004).

Cognitive and Behavioral Outcomes

Epidemiological studies link early life exposure to neurotoxic environmental chemicals with increased risk of learning disabilities, attention deficit hyperactivity disorder, and behavioral dysregulation. While causation is multifactorial, environmental chemical exposure is recognized as a major contributor to neurodevelopmental disorders (Grandjean & Landrigan, 2014). Children exposed to fragranced products in homes, schools, and childcare environments may experience subtle cognitive effects that accumulate over time, including reduced attention span, impaired executive function, and emotional dysregulation.

Autism Spectrum and Neurodevelopmental Vulnerability

Autism spectrum disorders involve complex interactions between genetics and environment. While fragrance exposure is not identified as a sole cause, environmental endocrine disruptors and neurotoxicants are increasingly recognized as contributors to neurodevelopmental vulnerability. Research demonstrates that prenatal exposure to endocrine disrupting chemicals can influence social behavior, communication, and sensory processing, all core features affected in autism spectrum disorders (Swan et al., 2015).

Immature Detoxification Systems

Children have immature detoxification and elimination systems. Hepatic enzymes, renal clearance mechanisms, and antioxidant defenses develop gradually. As a result, children may retain neurotoxic chemicals longer and at higher relative concentrations than adults. This reduced detoxification capacity increases vulnerability to cumulative neurotoxic burden from repeated fragrance exposure.

School and Childcare Environments

Fragrance exposure is common in schools and childcare settings through cleaning products, air fresheners, personal care items, and fragranced teaching materials. These environments often involve prolonged indoor exposure with limited ventilation. Studies report increased headaches, attention difficulties, and respiratory symptoms in children exposed to fragranced environments, supporting the need for fragrance free policies in educational settings (Steinemann, 2018).

Long Term Implications

Early neurodevelopmental disruption may not manifest immediately. Reduced cognitive reserve, altered stress response, and sensory sensitivity may increase vulnerability to later neurological disorders, learning challenges, and mental health conditions. Because neurodevelopment sets the foundation for lifelong brain function, reducing avoidable chemical exposure during childhood represents a critical preventive strategy.

Conclusion

Children represent the most vulnerable population with respect to synthetic fragrance exposure. Through prenatal transfer, endocrine disruption, sensory overload, and immature detoxification systems, fragrance related chemicals can interfere with neurodevelopment during critical windows of growth. Recognizing fragrance exposure as a modifiable environmental risk factor offers a powerful opportunity to protect developing brains. Creating fragrance free homes, schools, and childcare environments supports healthy neurodevelopment and promotes long term cognitive and neurological resilience.

9. Fertility and Pregnancy

Fertility and healthy pregnancy depend on precise hormonal signaling, cellular communication, and tightly regulated developmental processes. Environmental exposures that interfere with these systems can impair reproductive function and influence pregnancy outcomes. Synthetic fragrance exposure introduces endocrine disrupting and bioaccumulative chemicals during periods when hormonal balance is essential, raising concerns for both fertility and fetal development.

Hormonal Regulation and Reproductive Health

Reproductive function is governed by coordinated signaling across the hypothalamic pituitary gonadal axis. Small disruptions in estrogen, progesterone, testosterone, thyroid hormone, or cortisol can alter ovulation, sperm production, implantation, and early embryonic development. Many fragrance related chemicals exhibit endocrine disrupting activity. Phthalates, synthetic musks, and phenolic compounds interfere with hormone synthesis, receptor binding, and metabolism (Diamanti Kandarakis et al., 2009). Because fragranced products are used daily, exposure patterns align with chronic low dose hormonal interference rather than isolated events.

Female Fertility

Female fertility depends on regular ovulation, adequate luteal phase function, and a receptive endometrial environment. Studies associate phthalate exposure with altered menstrual cycle length, anovulation, reduced ovarian reserve markers, and impaired fertility outcomes (Meeker et al., 2009). Endocrine disruption may also impair follicular development and oocyte quality through oxidative stress and mitochondrial dysfunction. These effects can reduce conception rates and increase the risk of early pregnancy loss.

Male Fertility

Male reproductive health is highly sensitive to environmental endocrine disruptors. Phthalates commonly used in fragrance fixation exhibit antiandrogenic effects that reduce testosterone synthesis and impair spermatogenesis. Epidemiological studies link phthalate exposure with decreased sperm concentration, reduced motility, abnormal morphology, and increased DNA fragmentation (Meeker et al., 2009). Because sperm production occurs continuously, chronic exposure may produce sustained fertility impairment.

Prenatal Exposure and Placental Transfer

Many fragrance related chemicals are lipophilic and readily cross the placenta. Biomonitoring studies detect phthalates and synthetic musks in amniotic fluid, umbilical cord blood, and placental tissue, confirming direct fetal exposure (Swan et al., 2015). The placenta does not function as an absolute barrier. Instead, it can concentrate certain chemicals, prolonging fetal exposure during critical periods of organogenesis and neurodevelopment.

Pregnancy Outcomes and Complications

Endocrine disrupting chemicals have been associated with adverse pregnancy outcomes including preterm birth, low birth weight, gestational hypertension, and altered fetal growth patterns. Disruption of thyroid hormone and cortisol signaling during pregnancy plays a central role in these outcomes (Boas et al., 2012). Oxidative stress induced by chemical exposure further contributes to placental dysfunction and inflammatory activation, increasing obstetric risk.

Neurodevelopmental and Lifelong Effects

Prenatal exposure does not end at birth. Hormonal and neurodevelopmental disruption during gestation may influence long term outcomes including cognitive function, behavioral regulation, metabolic health, and reproductive development in offspring. Research demonstrates associations between prenatal endocrine disruptor exposure and later neurodevelopmental challenges, highlighting the transgenerational impact of chemical exposure (Grandjean & Landrigan, 2014).

Assisted Reproductive Technology and Exposure Sensitivity

Individuals undergoing fertility treatment may be particularly vulnerable to environmental exposures. Oocyte quality, embryo viability, and implantation success are sensitive to hormonal and oxidative balance. Studies suggest that reducing exposure to endocrine disrupting chemicals during fertility treatment improves reproductive outcomes, underscoring the clinical relevance of environmental control.

Occupational and Household Exposure

Occupational exposure increases risk due to duration and intensity. Healthcare workers, salon professionals, cleaners, and service workers often experience sustained fragrance exposure. Household exposure further compounds risk through personal care products, laundry agents, and air fresheners. Pregnant individuals may be unaware of exposure sources, particularly when fragrance ingredients are undisclosed.

Preventive Opportunity

Fertility and pregnancy represent windows of heightened vulnerability but also opportunity. Reducing fragrance exposure before conception and throughout pregnancy offers a practical and low risk intervention to support hormonal balance and fetal development. Environmental modification complements medical care and empowers individuals to protect reproductive health proactively.

Conclusion

Synthetic fragrance exposure represents a significant and underrecognized risk factor for fertility impairment and adverse pregnancy outcomes. Through endocrine disruption, oxidative stress, and placental transfer, fragrance related chemicals can interfere with reproductive function and fetal development during critical periods. Recognizing fragrance exposure as a modifiable environmental risk empowers individuals and clinicians to support fertility and pregnancy outcomes beyond medical intervention alone. Reducing exposure represents a meaningful step toward protecting reproductive health and promoting healthy beginnings for future generations.

Regulation Failure

Synthetic fragrance exposure persists not because the science is unclear, but because regulatory systems have failed to keep pace with evidence. Despite decades of data documenting adverse health effects, fragrance ingredients remain largely unregulated, undisclosed, and untested for long term safety in real world conditions. This regulatory gap shifts the burden of protection away from manufacturers and onto individuals, families, and workers. Understanding how and why this failure occurred is essential to correcting it.

The Regulatory Gap

In many countries, including the United States, fragrance ingredients are regulated under outdated chemical safety frameworks. **These frameworks often assess single chemicals in isolation rather than complex mixtures used daily over a lifetime.** Fragrance formulations may contain dozens to hundreds of chemicals. Yet most have never been evaluated for chronic low dose exposure, cumulative effects, or vulnerable populations such as pregnant individuals, children, or those with chronic illness.

Trade Secret Protections

One of the most significant barriers to regulation is the use of trade secret protections. Fragrance formulations are frequently exempt from full ingredient disclosure, even on products that come into direct contact with skin or are inhaled daily. As a result, consumers, clinicians, and researchers are often unable to identify specific exposure sources. This lack of transparency prevents informed decision making and limits the ability to conduct comprehensive health risk assessments.

Inadequate Safety Testing

Many fragrance ingredients entered the market decades ago under grandfathered status, meaning they were never required to undergo modern safety testing. Current regulatory standards often rely on industry submitted data, short term toxicity endpoints, and assumptions about safe exposure that do not reflect real world use patterns. These standards rarely account for cumulative exposure across multiple products or combined exposure to other environmental chemicals.

Voluntary Industry Oversight

In the absence of robust regulation, fragrance safety is often governed by voluntary industry organizations. While these bodies establish guidelines, they are not independent regulatory authorities and do not prioritize public health protection over commercial interests. Voluntary compliance lacks enforcement power and transparency. This model places consumer safety at the discretion of manufacturers rather than under enforceable public health standards.

Vulnerable Populations Left Unprotected

Regulatory frameworks frequently fail to account for populations with heightened vulnerability. Children, pregnant individuals, workers in high exposure occupations, and people with asthma, migraines, autoimmune disease, or neurological disorders face disproportionate risk. Without mandatory protections, these individuals are often forced to self regulate exposure in environments they cannot fully control.

International Inconsistencies

Regulation of fragrance chemicals varies widely across countries. Some regions restrict or ban specific compounds based on emerging evidence, while others continue unrestricted use. These inconsistencies underscore the absence of global consensus and highlight the influence of economic priorities over health based standards.

The Cost of Regulatory Failure

The consequences of regulatory inaction extend beyond individual symptoms. Fragrance related illness contributes to lost productivity, increased healthcare utilization, reduced quality of life, and workplace disability. When exposure is normalized and health effects are dismissed, individuals are often misdiagnosed, undertreated, or told symptoms are psychosomatic. This compounds harm and delays appropriate intervention.

Advocacy as a Public Health Tool

In the absence of adequate regulation, advocacy becomes a necessary component of protection. Advocacy does not require confrontation. It requires clarity, consistency, and evidence-based communication. Individuals can advocate by choosing fragrance-free products, sharing credible information, and requesting accommodations in workplaces, schools, and healthcare settings. Healthcare providers can advocate by recognizing fragrance exposure as a legitimate health risk, documenting symptoms, and supporting patients who request environmental modifications.

Readers are encouraged to share this book with legislators, workplace management, and human resources departments. It was intentionally designed and extensively researched to serve as an evidence-informed resource in professional and policy settings. The scientific data presented throughout can assist decision-makers in understanding the documented risks associated with fragrance exposure and in implementing protective policies grounded in established research.

Policy and Workplace Advocacy

Organizations can implement fragrance free policies that protect employees and visitors without compromising professionalism or hygiene. Evidence shows these policies reduce symptom burden and improve indoor air quality. Policymakers can strengthen chemical safety laws by requiring full ingredient disclosure, cumulative risk assessment, and independent safety testing. Advocacy at the policy level is essential for systemic change.

Building Momentum for Change

Public awareness has driven progress in areas such as smoking restrictions, lead removal, and asbestos regulation. Fragrance exposure represents a similar public health issue that requires sustained attention. Change occurs when evidence is communicated clearly, when affected individuals are believed, and when health is prioritized over convenience.

A Call to Action

For readers in the United States, awareness must lead to action.

Change does not begin with corporations or regulatory agencies. It begins with informed citizens who document harm, raise concerns, and insist on safer environments. Fragrance free policies exist in other countries because individuals spoke clearly and persistently, supported by scientific evidence and lived experience (Steinemann, 2016).

Readers are strongly encouraged to <u>send a copy of this book</u> to their local and state legislators, healthcare facility administrators, hospital systems, school boards, and workplace leadership. This book was intentionally written with peer reviewed studies and references included in every section so that concerns are not dismissed as personal preference or anecdotal experience. The evidence is provided to support meaningful dialogue and policy consideration.

Sharing personal experiences alongside documented research helps decision makers understand both the human impact and the scientific basis for change. Healthcare settings should lead this effort. Patients are already vulnerable, and unnecessary chemical exposure should never compromise safety, access to care, or health outcomes.

Progress begins when evidence is placed directly into the hands of those with the authority to act.

Conclusion

The continued widespread exposure to synthetic fragrance reflects a failure of regulation rather than a lack of scientific evidence. Trade secret protections, inadequate testing, and voluntary oversight have left consumers and workers without meaningful protection. Advocacy bridges this gap. Through informed choices, workplace initiatives, clinical recognition, and policy reform, it is possible to reduce exposure and protect public health. Regulation may lag, but awareness and action do not have to.

Fragrance Free Nations

Fragrance Free Nations: What the World Already Knows

Around the world, governments and healthcare systems have quietly acknowledged a truth that many individuals experience daily but struggle to name: fragranced environments can cause real harm. While fragrance products are marketed as symbols of cleanliness, wellness, and self expression, scientific and public health evidence has driven multiple countries to implement fragrance free policies in healthcare settings, government buildings, schools, and workplaces (Steinemann, 2016; Caress & Steinemann, 2009).

These policies are not cultural trends or personal preferences. They are responses to documented health risks, accessibility concerns, and occupational safety obligations. **Examining where these policies exist and why they were implemented reveals a growing international consensus that contrasts sharply with the limited protections found in the United States.**

Canada: A Global Leader in Fragrance Free Policy

Canada is widely recognized as the most advanced country in adopting fragrance free environments.

Fragrance free policies are implemented across federal government buildings, provincial health authorities, hospitals, clinics, schools, and public service workplaces. Many Canadian hospitals clearly state that staff, patients, and visitors are expected to avoid wearing scented products (Health Canada, 2018).

The rationale is grounded in public health. Canadian agencies acknowledge that fragranced products can trigger asthma attacks, migraines, respiratory distress, skin reactions, and neurological symptoms. **Fragrance sensitivity is treated as an accessibility and occupational health issue rather than a personal inconvenience** (Canadian Centre for Occupational Health and Safety [CCOHS], 2019).

Implementation began in the late 1990s and expanded significantly in the early 2000s alongside advances in indoor air quality research and disability inclusion standards. Today, fragrance free environments are considered a reasonable and necessary accommodation in public institutions.

Australia: Occupational Health and Safety in Practice

Australia has adopted fragrance free policies primarily through occupational health and safety frameworks.

Hospitals, healthcare clinics, and government agencies commonly maintain scent free guidelines that apply to employees and visitors. These policies are enforced internally as part of employer obligations to provide safe working environments (Safe Work Australia, 2020).

Australian authorities recognize that fragranced products contribute to respiratory illness, headaches, and chemical sensitivity among healthcare workers and patients. Rather than framing fragrance exposure as a lifestyle issue, it is treated as a workplace hazard similar to chemical cleaners or indoor pollutants (Steinemann, 2018).

United Kingdom: Patient Safety Comes First

The United Kingdom does not have a nationwide fragrance ban, but fragrance free expectations are common throughout National Health Service hospitals and clinics.

Many NHS facilities post signage requesting that patients, visitors, and staff refrain from wearing perfumes or scented products. Local councils and public buildings frequently adopt similar policies (NHS England, 2019).

These measures emerged in the early 2000s as part of patient safety initiatives, particularly for individuals with asthma, chronic respiratory disease, and migraines. Evidence shows that fragranced environments can worsen symptoms and interfere with clinical care (Caress & Steinemann, 2009).

Sweden and the Nordic Model of Prevention

Sweden and other Nordic countries have normalized fragrance free environments in healthcare, schools, and government buildings.

These policies align with a preventive public health philosophy that prioritizes environmental safety and chemical exposure reduction. Fragrance restrictions are widely accepted because chemical sensitivity and environmental illness are recognized as legitimate health conditions (Azuma et al., 2015).

Implementation in Nordic countries dates back several decades and is supported by strong environmental health regulations and precautionary principles.

Germany and France: Regulating the Chemicals Themselves

Germany and France focus heavily on regulating the chemical composition of fragranced products.

While fragrance free policies are not universally mandated, healthcare settings and workplaces often restrict fragrance use under occupational health laws. These countries enforce strict chemical labeling requirements and limit exposure to allergens, endocrine disrupting compounds, and volatile organic compounds (European Chemicals Agency, 2021).

Their regulatory approach reflects a precautionary model in which uncertain chemical safety justifies exposure reduction rather than assumed safety.

The United States: Policies Without Protection

The United States lacks a national fragrance free law. Restrictions exist only through internal policies within select federal agencies, hospitals, universities, and workplaces.

Some institutions discourage or prohibit fragrance use, but these measures are inconsistent and largely unenforceable beyond individual organizations. In the U.S., fragrance sensitivity is typically addressed only after harm occurs, framed as a disability accommodation rather than a preventable public health issue (U.S. Access Board, 2020).

This approach shifts responsibility onto affected individuals rather than institutions.

A Call to Action for American Readers

For readers in the United States, awareness must lead to action.

Change does not begin with corporations or regulatory agencies. It begins with informed citizens who document harm, raise concerns, and insist on safer environments. Fragrance free policies exist in other countries because individuals spoke clearly and persistently, supported by scientific evidence and lived experience (Steinemann, 2016).

Readers are strongly encouraged to <u>send a copy of this book </u>to their local and state legislators, healthcare facility administrators, hospital systems, school boards, and workplace leadership. This book was intentionally written with peer reviewed studies and references included in every section so that concerns are not dismissed as personal preference or anecdotal experience. The evidence is provided to support meaningful dialogue and policy consideration.

Sharing personal experiences alongside documented research helps decision makers understand both the human impact and the scientific basis for change. Healthcare settings should lead this effort. Patients are already vulnerable, and unnecessary chemical exposure should never compromise safety, access to care, or health outcomes.

Progress begins when evidence is placed directly into the hands of those with the authority to act.

The Global Pattern Is Clear

Across countries and healthcare systems, the same conclusion emerges. Fragrance free environments reduce harm, improve accessibility, and protect public health. The question is no longer whether fragranced products can cause injury. The evidence has already answered that. The remaining question is how long some nations will delay meaningful action.

Advocacy Insert

Advocacy Insert

How to Use This Book to Create Change

This book was written not only to inform, but to protect public health.

If you are reading *Killed by Fragrance*, you may already know firsthand that fragranced environments can cause real and sometimes severe health reactions. What many decision makers do not realize is that these reactions are not rare, subjective, or unsupported by evidence.

This book was intentionally structured to help bridge that gap.

Why This Book Matters to Policymakers and Administrators

Scientific research shows that approximately one third of adults report adverse health effects from fragranced products. These effects include migraines, asthma attacks, respiratory distress, neurological symptoms, skin reactions, and allergic responses. Despite this, fragranced products remain largely unregulated in public and healthcare settings.

Unlike personal testimonies alone, this book combines lived experience with peer reviewed research. Every major section includes scientific references so concerns cannot be dismissed as opinion, preference, or anecdote. The evidence presented reflects findings already recognized in other countries that have implemented fragrance free policies in healthcare, government, and public institutions.

Who Should Receive This Book

You are encouraged to share this book with individuals who have the authority to influence policy or workplace practices, including:

• Local and state legislators
• Healthcare facility administrators and hospital leadership
• Public health officials
• School board members and university administrators
• Workplace leadership and human resource departments

- Healthcare settings are especially important. Patients are already vulnerable, and unnecessary chemical exposure should never compromise safety, access to care, or health outcomes.

How to Use This Book Effectively

When sharing this book, consider including a short personal note explaining why fragrance exposure matters to you. Personal experience combined with scientific evidence is powerful.

Encourage recipients to review the referenced studies included throughout the book. These studies demonstrate that fragrance related illness is widespread, measurable, and preventable.

Ask a simple question:
What steps can be taken to reduce unnecessary fragrance exposure in public or healthcare environments?

Change does not require immediate legislation. Many countries and institutions began with fragrance free policies, signage, and indoor air quality standards. Awareness is the first step, but action must follow.

A Final Encouragement

Progress happens when evidence is placed directly into the hands of those who can act. By sharing this book, you are helping ensure that public health decisions are informed by science, compassion, and lived reality. Your voice matters. Your experience matters. And the evidence is now undeniable.

Contact Your Legislators and Advocate for Change

Use the link provided or scan the QR code below to visit https://www.usa.gov/elected-officials, where you can quickly identify your local, state, and federal legislators by entering your ZIP code. This official government resource makes it easy to determine the individuals responsible for shaping public health policy in your area. I encourage you to send them a copy of *Killed by Fragrance*, along with a brief note explaining why this issue matters to you personally. The evidence presented throughout this book demonstrates that fragrance exposure represents a significant and preventable public health concern. Informed leadership is essential to achieving meaningful and lasting policy change.

Short Letter to Include When Mailing *Killed by Fragrance*

Dear [Title and Name],

I am sharing this book, *Killed by Fragrance*, because fragrance exposure is a serious and underrecognized public health issue that affects millions of people, including myself or those I care about.

Scientific research shows that approximately one third of adults experience adverse health effects from fragranced products, including migraines, asthma, respiratory distress, and neurological symptoms. These reactions are not rare, imagined, or isolated. They are documented, preventable, and increasingly recognized in other countries through fragrance free policies in healthcare and public settings.

This book includes peer reviewed studies and references throughout to support the need for awareness and action. My hope is that it will encourage thoughtful consideration of fragrance free policies, particularly in healthcare and public environments where safety and accessibility should be paramount.

Thank you for taking the time to review this information and for your commitment to protecting public health.

Respectfully,
[Your Name]
[City and State, optional]

Healing After Exposure

Healing After Exposure

Reducing or eliminating exposure to synthetic fragrance is the first and most important step toward recovery. However, for many individuals, symptoms do not resolve immediately once exposure ends. This does not indicate permanent damage. It reflects the time required for biological systems to recalibrate after prolonged chemical stress. Healing after exposure is not random. It follows predictable physiological principles that involve nervous system regulation, inflammation control, endocrine balance, and effective detoxification. Within this framework, nutrition is not supportive. It is foundational.

Healing Requires a Structured Framework

Chronic fragrance exposure places sustained stress on detoxification pathways, hormonal signaling, immune regulation, and neurological processing. Over time, this burden may impair the body's ability to clear chemicals efficiently. Recovery requires more than simply avoiding fragrance. It requires restoring the internal environment that allows detoxification systems to function properly. This is where a structured nutritional framework becomes essential.

The ASTR Diet as the Foundation for Detoxification

The ASTR Diet, detailed in the book *Eat to Heal*, provides the nutritional foundation for safe and effective detoxification after chemical exposure.

ASTR is an acronym that reflects the four pillars required for healing.

A Anti inflammatory
Reduces systemic inflammation that interferes with detox enzyme function, hormone signaling, and nervous system regulation.

S Sustainable
Ensures detoxification strategies can be maintained long term without nutrient depletion or metabolic stress.

T Toxin free
Eliminates dietary sources of chemical burden including additives, preservatives,

pesticides, and ultra processed foods that compete with detoxification pathways.

R Restorative
Provides adequate macronutrients, micronutrients, and energy to support liver function, mitochondrial health, and cellular repair.

This framework avoids extreme restriction and instead restores metabolic capacity so detoxification can occur naturally and efficiently.

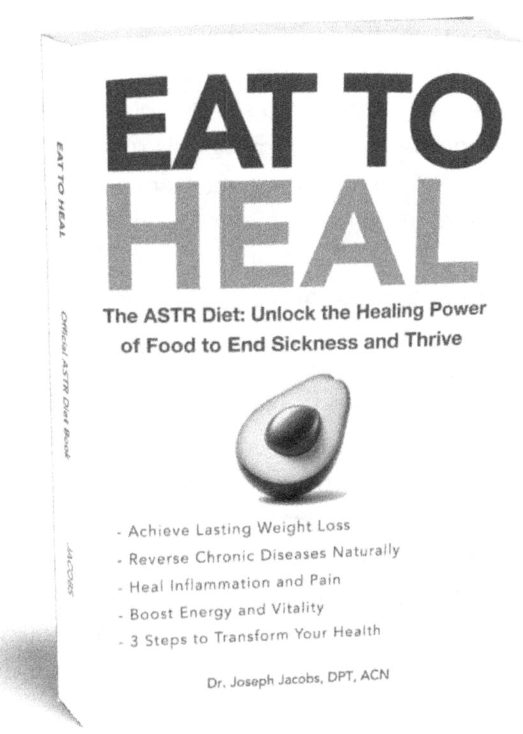

Detoxification Is Continuous, Not a One Time Event

Environmental exposure does not end. Even with reduced fragrance use, low level chemical exposure continues through air, water, and everyday consumer products. Because exposure is ongoing, the body's detoxification systems must function consistently, not intermittently. Within the ASTR framework, detoxification is not treated as a short term cleanse or aggressive intervention. It is supported daily through sustainable, whole food nutrition that nourishes the liver, kidneys, gastrointestinal tract, lymphatic system, and cellular antioxidant pathways throughout the year.

The ASTR Diet is intentionally designed to be sustainable for long term use. It is not restrictive, extreme, or cyclical. By emphasizing anti inflammatory nutrition, toxin conscious sourcing, balanced macronutrients, adequate protein, fiber, and micronutrient density, the diet continuously supports the body's natural elimination pathways. Rather than relying on periodic detox programs, the ASTR approach strengthens endogenous detox mechanisms through metabolic stability, blood sugar regulation, digestive efficiency, and cellular repair processes. Because the diet is balanced and sustainable, it can be maintained long term without nutrient depletion or hormonal disruption. Detoxification is not an event. It is a function. When nutrition consistently supports physiological balance, detox pathways operate efficiently year round.

The Role of Clinical Nutrition and Laboratory Guidance

Detoxification should never be based on guesswork. Generic detox programs do not account for individual differences in liver enzyme activity, nutrient status, inflammatory load, or hormonal balance. The safest and most effective approach is to work with a **clinical nutritionist who has specialized training in detoxification and functional assessment**. This professional evaluates laboratory data such as liver function markers, nutrient deficiencies, inflammatory indicators, metabolic markers, and hormone balance. Lab guided detoxification allows interventions to be precise rather than indiscriminate. This approach prevents overloading detox pathways, avoids nutrient depletion, and reduces the risk of symptom flares.

Why Commercial Detox Programs Often Fail

Many commercial detox programs rely on extreme calorie restriction, liquid fasting, excessive supplementation, or unsupported claims. These approaches can impair detoxification rather than support it. Inadequate protein intake, insufficient minerals, and poor blood sugar regulation reduce the liver's ability to perform phase one and phase two detoxification. Within the ASTR framework, detoxification is never separated from metabolic stability.

Supporting Detoxification Within the ASTR Framework

Detoxification is supported through:

- Adequate protein intake to supply amino acids required for detox enzyme function
- Fiber rich foods to support gastrointestinal elimination
- Hydration to assist renal clearance
- Anti inflammatory nutrients to reduce oxidative stress
- Stable blood sugar to prevent cortisol driven detox impairment
- Supplementation is only introduced when indicated by laboratory data and under professional supervision. Supplements should not be taken without medical oversight, as excessive or inappropriate use can worsen symptoms and strain detox organs.

Nervous System and Hormonal Recovery

Detoxification is impaired when the nervous system is dysregulated. Chronic stress, poor sleep, and sensory overload reduce detox efficiency. The ASTR framework emphasizes sleep consistency, circadian alignment, stress regulation, and gentle movement to restore autonomic balance. Hormonal recovery is supported through regular meals, nutrient adequacy, and avoidance of metabolic stressors.

Sensory and Symptom Recalibration

Heightened sensitivity after fragrance exposure reflects nervous system sensitization rather than permanent injury. As inflammation decreases and detoxification improves, sensory thresholds often normalize. Progress is gradual. Temporary symptom fluctuations during detox phases are possible and should be interpreted as signals to adjust intensity, not push harder.

Timeline and Expectations

Healing timelines vary. Some individuals experience improvement within weeks, while others require months of structured support. Within the ASTR framework, progress is measured by improved tolerance, reduced symptom frequency, increased energy, and improved laboratory markers rather than speed alone.

Conclusion

Healing after synthetic fragrance exposure requires more than avoidance. It requires restoring the internal environment that allows detoxification, regulation, and repair to occur. The ASTR Diet provides a structured, science based nutritional framework that supports detoxification safely and sustainably. When paired with **lab guided clinical nutrition oversight**, detoxification becomes a precise therapeutic tool rather than a guessing game. Detoxification support throughout the year, guided by laboratory data and grounded in the ASTR principles of anti inflammatory, sustainable, toxin free, and restorative nutrition, offers the most effective path toward recovery. When exposure is reduced and the body is properly supported, healing is not forced. It unfolds.

Safer Alternatives

Reducing exposure to synthetic fragrance does not require expensive specialty products, complicated routines, or significant time investment. In fact, homemade fragrance free cleaning solutions are among the most affordable, effective, and health conscious options available. With only a few basic ingredients and reusable containers, most households can replace dozens of fragranced products quickly and permanently. This chapter focuses on practical, evidence supported alternatives that are easy to implement, cost effective, and realistic for everyday life. These solutions prioritize health protection while maintaining effective cleanliness.

Why Homemade Cleaners Are a Better Option

Homemade fragrance free cleaners offer several advantages over commercial fragranced products.

- They are significantly cheaper. A single bulk purchase of baking soda, white vinegar, and alcohol can replace multiple specialized cleaners and last for months.
- They are healthier. These ingredients clean effectively without releasing synthetic fragrance chemicals into indoor air or leaving residues on skin, clothing, or household surfaces.
- They are efficient. Most recipes take less than one minute to prepare and can be reused indefinitely with refillable containers.
- They simplify the home. Instead of managing numerous specialized products, a small number of versatile solutions meet nearly all household cleaning needs.

What You Need to Get Started

Creating a fragrance free cleaning system requires only a few basic items.

- White distilled vinegar
- Baking soda
- Seventy percent isopropyl alcohol
- Water
- Reusable spray bottles and small containers

Once these items are available, most routine household cleaning needs are fully covered without additional purchases.

Understanding Product Labels

Products labeled unscented may still contain fragrance chemicals used to mask odor. These compounds can off gas into indoor air even when no scent is consciously detected. Products labeled fragrance free are intended to exclude fragrance ingredients, but labeling standards vary and disclosure is not always complete. Homemade single ingredient solutions eliminate this uncertainty and provide full control over exposure.

The Science Behind Safer Cleaning Ingredients

Homemade cleaners are often dismissed as less effective than commercial products, yet research demonstrates that vinegar, alcohol, and baking soda are highly effective for routine household cleaning and sanitation when used appropriately.

White Vinegar (Acetic Acid)

White distilled vinegar contains approximately 4 to 6 percent acetic acid, which has well documented antimicrobial properties. Laboratory studies show that acetic acid effectively reduces populations of common household pathogens, including Escherichia coli, Salmonella, Listeria monocytogenes, and Staphylococcus aureus on hard surfaces (Entani et al., 1998). Acetic acid disrupts bacterial cell membranes and interferes with metabolic function, contributing to microbial inactivation (Johnston & Gaas, 2006). In addition to its antimicrobial effects, vinegar dissolves mineral deposits, soap scum, and grease, making it effective for kitchens, bathrooms, glass, and appliances (Rutala & Weber, 2016). While vinegar is not classified as a hospital grade disinfectant, evidence supports its use for low risk household sanitation without introducing volatile fragrance chemicals into indoor environments.

Alcohol (Seventy Percent Isopropyl or Ethanol)

Alcohol based cleaners are widely recognized for rapid antimicrobial activity. Research consistently demonstrates that alcohol concentrations between 60 and 80 percent are optimal for protein denaturation and disruption of lipid membranes in bacteria and enveloped viruses (Kampf, 2018). Seventy percent isopropyl alcohol has been shown to rapidly inactivate influenza viruses, coronaviruses, Staphylococcus aureus, and Pseudomonas aeruginosa, often within seconds of contact (McDonnell & Russell, 1999). Because alcohol evaporates quickly, it leaves no residue and does not require rinsing on non food surfaces. These properties make alcohol particularly effective for high touch surfaces such as doorknobs, light switches, phones, remote controls, and electronics.

Baking Soda (Sodium Bicarbonate)

Baking soda functions as a mild abrasive, deodorizer, and pH buffering agent. Its fine crystalline structure allows effective mechanical removal of grime without scratching most household surfaces (U.S. Environmental Protection Agency, 2021). Research shows that sodium bicarbonate neutralizes acidic odors and improves cleaning efficiency by facilitating physical removal of organic material and surface debris that can harbor microorganisms (Farmer et al., 2013). While baking soda is not a disinfectant, it enhances overall cleanliness and reduces odor without masking smells with fragrance compounds.

Comparison With Commercial Fragranced Cleaners

Studies examining indoor air quality consistently demonstrate that fragranced cleaning products emit volatile organic compounds, including terpenes that can react with ozone to form secondary pollutants such as formaldehyde (Nazaroff & Weschler, 2004). These emissions occur even in products marketed as green or natural. In contrast, single ingredient cleaners such as vinegar, alcohol, and baking soda do not release synthetic fragrance compounds or persistent indoor air pollutants. This significantly reduces inhalation exposure, particularly for children, pregnant individuals, and those with asthma, migraines, or chemical sensitivity (Steinemann et al., 2017).

Simplifying Personal Care Exposure

Personal care products are a major source of daily fragrance exposure due to repeated skin contact and inhalation. Choosing fragrance free soaps, shampoos, lotions, deodorants, and cosmetics with minimal ingredients reduces cumulative chemical burden. Cleanliness does not require scent. In many individuals, skin health improves when unnecessary additives are removed. It is important to recognize that natural does not always mean safe. **Essential oils are volatile compounds and may trigger neurological, respiratory, or allergic symptoms in sensitive individuals**. For many people, truly fragrance free options represent the safest choice.

Conclusion

Homemade fragrance free cleaners are safer, more affordable, and easier to maintain than commercial fragranced products. With vinegar, baking soda, alcohol, and a few reusable bottles, most households can significantly reduce chemical exposure while maintaining effective cleanliness. Fragrance free living is not extreme or inconvenient. It is practical, economical, and intentional. Small, informed changes meaningfully reduce cumulative exposure, support detoxification, and protect neurological, hormonal, respiratory, immune, and reproductive health.

Conclusion

Choosing Health in a Fragranced World

Synthetic fragrance has become deeply embedded in modern life to the point that its presence is rarely examined. It permeates products marketed as clean, soothing, luxurious, and safe. Its ubiquity has normalized exposure and obscured scrutiny. Yet the scientific evidence presented throughout this book makes one fact unmistakable: fragrance is not biologically neutral. It is a chemically complex, bioactive mixture capable of influencing neurological, hormonal, respiratory, immune, reproductive, and developmental systems. What makes this reality both urgent and empowering is that most fragrance exposure is voluntary. Unlike many environmental hazards that are difficult to control, fragranced consumer products are discretionary. They are added for sensory appeal, not necessity. This means exposure can be meaningfully reduced through informed, intentional decisions.

Change does not require alarmism, perfection, or extreme lifestyle disruption. It requires awareness. It requires recognizing that "fragrance" on a label represents more than scent. It represents chemical exposure. Once that distinction is understood, action becomes straightforward.

A Practical Call to Action

The path forward begins simply.

- Take the shopping checklist provided in this book with you the next time you shop. Purchase bulk baking soda, white distilled vinegar, 70 percent isopropyl alcohol, fragrance free detergent, wool dryer balls, and a few reusable spray bottles and containers.
- Once these items are in your home, you are equipped to replace the majority of fragranced cleaning and laundry products in your environment.
- Set aside one short window of time. In less than fifteen minutes, you can prepare every cleaning solution outlined in this book, pour them into containers, and label them clearly. There is no ongoing mixing, no daily effort, and no complicated process. Once complete, your home is stocked with safer, effective alternatives that will last for months.

- This single step eliminates repeated shopping for fragranced products and removes a constant source of unnecessary chemical exposure from your living space.

The Power of Small, Consistent Choices

Health is not restored through a single dramatic action. It is built through small, consistent decisions that reduce burden and support balance. Throwing out fragranced cleaners, air fresheners, fabric softeners, and dryer sheets is not wasteful. It is intentional. Replacing them with simple, fragrance free solutions reduces cumulative exposure and protects the systems that allow the body to function optimally. Clean does not require scent. Comfort does not require chemicals. Safety does not require compromise.

Protecting the Most Vulnerable

Reducing fragrance exposure is especially important during pregnancy, infancy, childhood, and periods of illness. These life stages represent windows of heightened sensitivity, but also windows of opportunity. By creating fragrance free environments, you protect neurological development, hormonal signaling, immune resilience, and long term health not only for yourself, but for those who depend on you.

A Shift in Perspective

Fragrance free living is not about restriction. It is about clarity. It is the decision to remove what is unnecessary so the body can do what it is designed to do. Regulate. Repair. Heal. This approach does not require perfection. It requires intention. Every product replaced reduces exposure. Every informed choice strengthens resilience.

Moving Forward

As you move forward, let this book serve as a reference rather than a rulebook. Return to the shopping list when needed. Share the recipes with others. Advocate for fragrance free spaces where possible. Speak calmly and confidently about your choices. Most importantly, trust your body's ability to respond when unnecessary chemical burden is removed. The air in your home matters. The products you touch matter. The choices you make daily matter. Throw out what no longer serves your health. Take your shopping list with you. Set aside fifteen minutes. Label your containers. Then live in a space that supports healing rather than hinders it. This is not an extreme choice. It is a wise one. And it begins today.

Recipes

Effective household cleaning does not require fragrance or harsh chemicals. The following fragrance free solutions are simple to prepare, quick to use, and supported by evidence for routine household cleaning and sanitation.

Glass and Mirror Cleaner

Use for: Windows, mirrors, and glass surfaces
Ingredients
- One cup water
- One cup white vinegar

Directions
Combine ingredients in a spray bottle. Spray lightly onto the surface and wipe with a microfiber cloth or newspaper to remove streaks and residue.

General Counter and Surface Cleaner

Use for: Kitchen counters, bathroom surfaces, sealed countertops, and appliances
Ingredients
- One cup water
- One half cup white vinegar

Directions
Spray onto the surface and wipe with a clean cloth.
Important note:
Do not use vinegar on natural stone such as granite or marble. For stone surfaces, use water with a small amount of unscented liquid soap.

All Purpose Everyday Cleaner

Use for: Routine cleaning of most sealed household surfaces
Ingredients
- Two cups water
- One tablespoon white vinegar
- One teaspoon unscented liquid soap

Directions
Mix gently in a spray bottle. Shake lightly before each use. Wipe surfaces with a clean cloth.

Baking Soda Scrub

Use for: Sinks, tubs, stovetops, and soap residue
Ingredients
• Baking soda
• Water to form a paste
Directions
Apply the paste to the surface. Allow it to sit for five to ten minutes, scrub gently, and rinse thoroughly.

Toilet Bowl Cleaner

Use for: Basic cleaning and deodorizing
Ingredients
• One cup baking soda
• One cup white vinegar
Directions
Add baking soda to the toilet bowl, followed by vinegar. Allow the mixture to foam for ten minutes, scrub with a toilet brush, and flush.

Sanitizing With Alcohol

Use for: High touch surfaces such as doorknobs, light switches, phones, and remote controls
Ingredient
• Seventy percent isopropyl alcohol
Directions
Apply lightly to a clean cloth or directly to the surface. Allow to air dry.
Safety note:
Ensure adequate ventilation and do not mix alcohol with other cleaning agents.

Refrigerator and Microwave Cleaner

Use for: Food contact surfaces
Ingredients
• One cup warm water

• One tablespoon baking soda
Directions
Wipe surfaces with a clean cloth dipped in the solution. This removes residue and neutralizes odors without fragrance.

Drain Freshening

Use for: Mild drain odor control
Ingredients
• One half cup baking soda
• One cup white vinegar
• Hot water
Directions
Pour baking soda into the drain, followed by vinegar. Allow the mixture to foam for five minutes, then flush with hot water.

Fragrance Free Laundry Care

Laundry products are a major source of prolonged fragrance exposure because scent compounds bind to fabric and continue to off gas over time. Use fragrance free detergent only. Eliminate fabric softeners and dryer sheets entirely.

Replacing Fabric Softener and Dryer Sheets

Use wool dryer balls instead. Wool dryer balls soften clothing, reduce static, improve airflow in the dryer, and shorten drying time without coating fabrics in chemicals. Use three to six dryer balls per load, depending on load size. Dryer balls are reusable for hundreds of loads and safe for sensitive skin.

Improving Indoor Air Quality

Remove continuous fragrance sources such as air fresheners, plug ins, scented candles, and incense. Ventilate the home regularly when weather permits. Vacuum and dust frequently to remove fragrance compounds that bind to household surfaces. Use high quality air filtration when needed.

Shopping Checklist

This checklist is designed to replace dozens of fragranced products with a small number of affordable, effective essentials. Most items are purchased once in bulk and last for months.

Essential Ingredients
- White distilled vinegar
- Baking soda
- 70 percent isopropyl alcohol
- Unscented liquid soap or castile soap
- Clean water

Laundry Essentials
- Fragrance free laundry detergent
- Wool dryer balls

Tools and Containers
- Reusable spray bottles
- Small storage containers or jars
- Microfiber cloths or cotton cleaning cloths
- Scrub brush or sponge

Optional Support Items
- High quality air filter
- Vacuum with HEPA filtration
- Glass spray bottle for alcohol based solutions
- Once these items are in place, nearly all household cleaning needs can be met without fragranced products.

Important Safety Notes
- Never mix vinegar with bleach
- Never mix alcohol with other cleaners
- Avoid vinegar on marble, granite, or natural stone
- Store all solutions out of reach of children

How to Access Online Content

1. Open the camera app on your smartphone.
2. Point the camera at the barcode.
3. A notification will appear with a link. Tap the notification to open the link in your browser.

Limited Time Offer: FREE 30-minute Health Coach Consultation

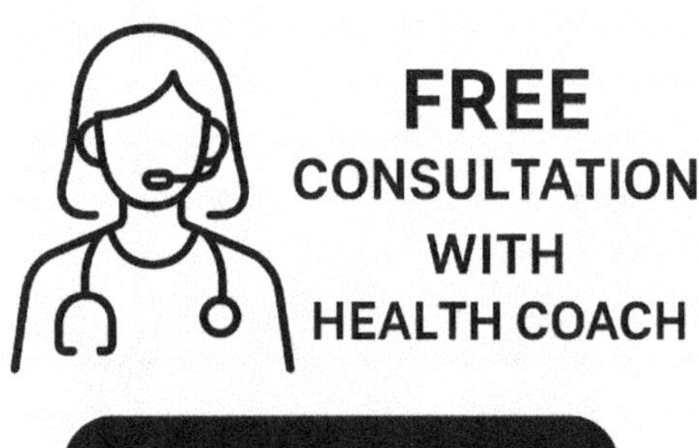

EAT TO HEAL
HEAL
The ASTR Diet: Unlock the Healing Power
of Food to End Sickness and Thrive

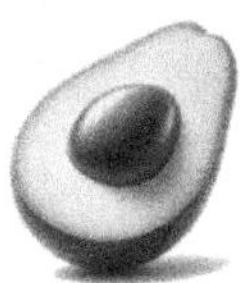

- Achieve Lasting Weight Loss
- Reverse Chronic Diseases Naturally
- Heal Inflammation and Pain
- Boost Energy and Vitality
- 3 Steps to Transform Your Health

Dr. Joseph Jacobs, DPT, ACN

EAT TO HEAL
Official ASTR Diet Book
JACOBS

PAIN
NO MORE
BOUNS VIDEOS
7 PROVEN SECRETS
TO END CHRONIC PAIN

- Stop Pain Before It's Too Late & End Pain For Good
- 45+ Studies Reveal The Secrets of Effective Pain Relief
- Secrets That Could Save You $1000s
- 21 Medical Myths Debunked: What Your Doctor Got Wrong

Dr. Joseph Jacobs, DPT, ACN

PAIN NO MORE
7 PROVEN SECRETS TO END CHRONIC PAIN
JACOBS

REVERSING
DIABETES

10 NATURAL SECRETS TO REVERSE DIABETES WITHOUT DRUGS

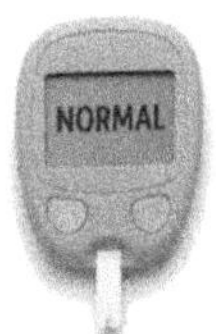

- Drug-Free, Side-Effect-Free, Science-Backed Healing
- Treat the Root Cause, Not Just the Symptoms
- Proven Natural Strategies That Get Results

Dr. Joseph Jacobs, DPT, ACN

REVERSING
HIGH BLOOD PRESSURE

7 NATURAL SECRETS TO SAFELY LOWER BLOOD PRESSURE

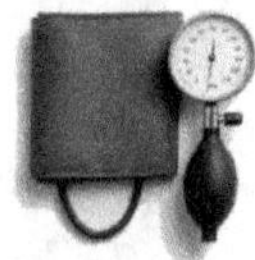

- Natural Solutions That Work
- Backed by Extensive Research
- Fix the Root Cause, Not Just the Numbers
- No Drugs, No Side Effects

Dr. Joseph Jacobs, DPT, ACN

BEATING ANXIETY & DEPRESSION

BONUS VIDEOS

14 NATURAL SECRETS TO A HAPPIER LIFE

- Conquer Anxiety & Depression Naturally
- Heal the Root Causes & Reclaim Your Life
- Created by a Doctor Who Conquered PTSD & Depression
- Science-Based Strategies for Lasting Change

Dr. Joseph Jacobs, DPT, ACN

BEATING MIGRAINES

BONUS VIDEOS

7 NATURAL SECRETS FOR LASTING RELIEF

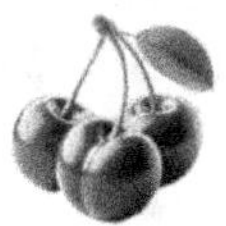

- End Migraines Naturally
- Clinically Proven Methods
- Treat the Root Cause, Not Symptoms
- Insights from a Doctor & Migraine Survivor
- Research-Backed Relief for Life

Dr. Joseph Jacobs, DPT, ACN

Your SHOES HURT YOU

Why Does Your Pain Keep Coming Back and *How to Fix It*

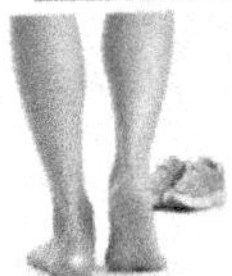

BONUS VIDEOS

- Fix Your Feet. Fix Your Pain.
- Why Modern Shoes Create Chronic Pain
- Backed by Biomechanics and Clinical Research

Dr. Joseph Jacobs, DPT, ACN

BEATING BACK PAIN

BONUS VIDEOS

7 NATURAL SECRETS FOR LASTING RELIEF

- End Back Pain Naturally
- Clinically Tested, Doctor-Approved
- Fix the Root Causes, Not Just Symptoms
- Backed by Science & Research
- Created by a Doctor Who Beat Chronic Pain

Dr. Joseph Jacobs, DPT, ACN

Glossary

Absorption: The process by which a substance enters the body through the skin, lungs, or digestive tract.

Acute Exposure: Short term exposure to a substance that occurs over a brief period and may cause immediate symptoms.

Allergen: A substance that triggers an immune response in sensitized individuals.

Allergic Contact Dermatitis: An immune mediated skin reaction caused by sensitization to a chemical allergen.

ASTR Diet: A clinical nutrition framework based on Anti inflammatory, Sustainable, Toxin free, and Restorative principles designed to support long term physiological resilience.

Autonomic Nervous System: The division of the nervous system that controls involuntary functions such as heart rate, digestion, breathing, and stress response.

Bioaccumulation: The gradual buildup of chemicals in the body when exposure exceeds elimination capacity.

Bioactive Mixture: A combination of chemical substances capable of interacting with and altering biological systems.

Biologically Neutral: A substance that produces no measurable physiological effect; synthetic fragrance does not meet this definition.

Blood Brain Barrier: A protective barrier that regulates which substances can pass from the bloodstream into the brain.

Bronchoconstriction: Narrowing of the airways that can cause wheezing, chest tightness, or shortness of breath.

Central Sensitization: A state in which the nervous system becomes hypersensitive and overreacts to stimuli that were previously tolerated.

Chemical Exposure: Contact with chemical substances through inhalation, skin absorption, or ingestion that may influence bodily function.

Chronic Exposure: Repeated or continuous exposure to a substance over long periods, often at low doses.

Cumulative Exposure: The total exposure to a chemical from multiple sources over time.

Cytokines: Immune signaling proteins that regulate inflammation and immune responses.

Dermal Absorption: The passage of chemicals through the skin into the bloodstream.

Detoxification: The body's natural process of neutralizing and eliminating toxins through organs such as the liver, kidneys, lungs, and gastrointestinal tract.

Discretionary Product: A consumer item used for preference or sensory enhancement rather than essential health or survival needs.

Endocrine Disrupting Chemicals (EDCs): Chemicals that interfere with hormone production, signaling, or metabolism.

Endocrine System: The network of glands and hormones that regulate metabolism, reproduction, stress response, growth, and overall physiological balance.

Environmental Exposure: Contact with substances present in air, water, food, or consumer products.

Environmental Load: The total cumulative burden of chemical exposures from all sources.

Fine and Ultrafine Particles: Microscopic airborne particles capable of penetrating deep into the lungs and entering the bloodstream.

Fragrance: A mixture of natural and synthetic chemicals added to products to create scent, often without full ingredient disclosure.

Fragrance Sensitivity: Adverse health reactions triggered by exposure to fragranced products.

Hormonal Dysregulation: Disruption of normal hormone levels or signaling within the body.

Immune Activation: Stimulation of immune pathways in response to perceived foreign substances.

Indoor Air Chemistry: Chemical reactions that occur between airborne substances inside buildings, sometimes forming secondary pollutants.

Indoor Air Quality: The condition of air inside buildings influenced by ventilation, pollutant emissions, and chemical reactions.

Inflammation: A biological response to stress or injury that can become harmful when chronic or dysregulated.

Inhalation Exposure: Entry of chemicals into the body through breathing.

Irritant Receptors: Sensory receptors that detect chemical or physical irritation and activate protective reflexes.

Liver Detoxification Pathways: Enzymatic systems that chemically modify substances to allow safe elimination from the body.

Low Dose Exposure: Exposure to small amounts of a chemical that may still produce biological effects over time.

Lymphatic System: A network of vessels and nodes that supports immune function and fluid balance.

Macrocyclic Musks: A newer class of synthetic fragrance compounds marketed as alternatives to older musk types.

Metabolic Stress: Physiological strain caused by inflammation, toxin exposure, or blood sugar instability.

Multiple Chemical Sensitivity (MCS): A condition marked by adverse reactions to low levels of common environmental chemicals.

Neurodevelopment: The growth and maturation of the brain and nervous system.

Neurological Activation: Stimulation of nerve pathways affecting mood, cognition, or sensory perception.

Neurotoxicity: Damage or dysfunction of the nervous system caused by toxic substances.

Occupational Exposure: Chemical exposure occurring as part of a work environment.

Olfactory System: The sensory system responsible for smell and its direct neurological connections to the limbic system.

Oxidative Stress: Cellular damage caused by an imbalance between free radicals and antioxidant defenses.

Parfum: A labeling term used interchangeably with fragrance that may represent numerous undisclosed chemicals.

Phase One Detoxification: The initial liver detox stage that chemically modifies substances.

Phase Two Detoxification: The liver detox stage that prepares modified substances for safe elimination.

Polycyclic Musks: Persistent synthetic fragrance compounds commonly detected in human tissue and environmental samples.

Reproductive Toxicity: Adverse effects on fertility, pregnancy, or fetal development.

Respiratory Irritation: Inflammation or discomfort in the airways following inhalation of irritants.

Secondary Pollutants: New chemicals formed when airborne substances react with one another in indoor environments.

Sensitization: A process in which repeated exposure lowers the threshold for reaction to a substance.

Sensory Processing: The nervous system's ability to receive and respond appropriately to sensory input.

Sympathetic Nervous System: The branch of the autonomic nervous system responsible for fight or flight stress responses.

Synthetic Fragrance: Artificial scent compounds often derived from petroleum based chemicals.

Synthetic Musk: A laboratory manufactured fragrance compound designed to create long lasting scent.

Thyroid Disruption: Interference with thyroid hormone production or signaling.

Toxic Load: The cumulative amount of toxic substances present in the body.

Toxicological Burden: The total physiological impact of chemical exposures over time.

Trigeminal Nerve: A cranial nerve that detects irritation, pain, and chemical stimuli in the face and airways.

Ultraviolet Radiation: Energy from sunlight that can interact with chemicals on the skin and influence biological effects.

Volatile Organic Compounds (VOCs): Chemicals that easily evaporate into the air and are commonly emitted by fragranced products.

Voluntary Exposure: Exposure resulting from personal product use rather than unavoidable environmental contamination.

References

1. Steinemann A. Fragranced consumer products: exposures and effects. *Air Qual Atmos Health*. 2016;9(5):835–847.
2. Steinemann A. Health and societal effects from exposure to fragranced consumer products. *Air Qual Atmos Health*. 2016;9:861–866.
3. Steinemann A. Fragranced consumer products and effects on health. *J Environ Health*. 2018;80(9):8–15.
4. Steinemann A, Klaschka U, Nematollahi N. Health effects from fragranced consumer products. *Air Qual Atmos Health*. 2019;12(6):719–727.
5. Steinemann A. Chemicals emitted from fragranced consumer products. *Environ Impact Assess Rev*. 2011;31(3):328–333.
6. Caress SM, Steinemann AC. Prevalence of fragrance sensitivity in the American population. *J Environ Health*. 2009;71(7):46–50.
7. Weschler CJ, Shields HC. Indoor ozone reactions with terpenes: secondary pollutant formation. *Atmos Environ*. 1997;31(21):3481–3492.
8. Nazaroff WW, Weschler CJ. Cleaning products and indoor air quality. *Atmos Environ*. 2004;38(18):2841–2865.
9. Singer BC, Destaillats H, Hodgson AT, Nazaroff WW. Cleaning products and secondary air pollutants. *Atmos Environ*. 2006;40(35):6696–6710.
10. Weschler CJ. Chemistry in indoor environments. *Chem Rev*. 2011;111(6):3884–3897.
11. Weschler CJ. Ozone in indoor environments. *Indoor Air*. 2006;16(4):269–288.
12. Weschler CJ. Changes in indoor pollutants since the 1950s. *Atmos Environ*. 2009;43(1):153–169.
13. Anderson RC, Anderson JH. Acute toxic effects of fragrance exposure. *Arch Environ Health*. 1998;53(2):138–146.
14. Ziem GE, McTamney J. Chemical injury and fragrance exposure. *Arch Environ Health*. 1997;52(5):322–329.
15. Doty RL. Olfaction. *Annu Rev Psychol*. 2001;52:423–452.
16. Doty RL, Deems DA, Stellar S. Olfactory and trigeminal influences on behavior. *Annu Rev Neurosci*. 2004;27:343–366.
17. Dalton P. Upper airway irritation and nervous system response. *Toxicol Sci*. 2003;74(1):1–8.
18. Kelman L. The triggers or precipitants of the migraine attack. *Headache*. 2007;47(5):772–777.
19. Burstein R, Noseda R, Borsook D. Migraine pathophysiology. *Neuron*. 2015;87(3):502–514.
20. Kilburn KH. Neurobehavioral impairment from chemical exposure. *Arch Environ Health*. 2000;55(1):11–17.
21. Bell IR, Miller CS, Schwartz GE. Neural sensitization and chemical intolerance. *Arch Environ Health*. 2001;56(6):504–517.
22. Grandjean P, Landrigan PJ. Neurotoxicity of industrial chemicals. *Lancet*. 2014;13(4):330–338.
23. Mendell MJ. Indoor environmental quality and health outcomes. *Indoor Air*. 2004;14(suppl 7):82–91.
24. Mølhave L. Sick building syndrome. *Indoor Air*. 2009;19(1):5–11.
25. Meeker JD, Sathyanarayana S, Swan SH. Phthalates and endocrine disruption. *Philos Trans R Soc Lond B Biol Sci*. 2009;364(1526):2097–2113.
26. Diamanti-Kandarakis E, et al. Endocrine disrupting chemicals. *Endocr Rev*. 2009;30(4):293–342.
27. Gore AC, Chappell VA, Fenton SE, et al. Endocrine Society scientific statement on endocrine disrupting chemicals. *Endocr Rev*. 2015;36(6):E1–E150.

References

28. Boas M, Feldt Rasmussen U, Main KM. Thyroid effects of endocrine disrupting chemicals. *Mol Cell Endocrinol.* 2012;355(2):240–248.

29. Swan SH, et al. Prenatal phthalate exposure and reproductive development. *Hum Reprod.* 2015;30(4):963–972.

30. Landrigan PJ, Goldman LR. Children's vulnerability to toxic chemicals. *Environ Health Perspect.* 2011;119(1):8–13.

31. Braun JM. Early life exposure to endocrine disrupting chemicals. *Curr Opin Pediatr.* 2017;29(2):243–250.

32. Reiner JL, Wong CM, Arcaro KF, Kannan K. Synthetic musks in human milk from the United States. *Environ Sci Technol.* 2007;41(11):3815–3820.

33. Basketter DA, et al. Fragrance allergens and skin sensitization. *Toxicol Appl Pharmacol.* 2019;362:114–120.

34. Kimber I, Basketter DA, Gerberick GF, Dearman RJ. Chemical sensitization and allergic contact dermatitis. *Chem Res Toxicol.* 2011;24(4):500–512.

35. Johansen JD, et al. Fragrance contact allergy. *Contact Dermatitis.* 2011;65(6):321–330.

36. Brown RP, Delp MD, Lindstedt SL, Rhomberg LR, Beliles RP. Physiological parameters for dermal absorption modeling. *Toxicol Ind Health.* 2013;29(1):1–40.

37. World Health Organization. *Dermal Exposure: Environmental Health Criteria 242.* Geneva, Switzerland: WHO; 2011.

38. Scientific Committee on Consumer Safety. *Guidance on Dermal Absorption.* European Commission; 2012.

39. Api AM, et al. Dermal absorption and phototoxicity of fragrance ingredients. *Food Chem Toxicol.* 2015;81:1–10.

40. International Agency for Research on Cancer. *IARC Monographs on the Evaluation of Carcinogenic Risks to Humans.* Lyon, France: IARC; 2012.

41. Kortenkamp A, Faust M. Regulating chemical mixtures. *Science.* 2018;361(6399):224–226.

42. Carpenter DO. Effects of persistent and bioaccumulative chemicals on human health. *Rev Environ Health.* 2011;26(2):103–115.

43. Lacour M, Zunder T, Schmidtke K, et al. Multiple chemical sensitivity syndrome. *Int J Hyg Environ Health.* 2005;208(3):141–151.

44. Pall ML. Elevated nitric oxide and peroxynitrite in multiple chemical sensitivity. *Med Hypotheses.* 2002;59(6):726–735.

45. Lan Q, Zhang L, Li G, et al. Hematotoxicity in workers exposed to low benzene levels. *Science.* 2004;306(5702):1774–1776.

46. Pezzoli G, Cereda E. Exposure to pesticides or solvents and Parkinson disease. *Neurology.* 2013;80(22):2035–2041.

47. Trasande L, et al. Chemical exposures and public health costs. *Lancet Planet Health.* 2016;1(1):e19–e27.

48. Tickner JA, et al. The precautionary principle in chemical policy. *Environ Health Perspect.* 2003;111(1):A56–A57.

49. U.S. Government Accountability Office. *Chemical Regulation: Observations on the Toxic Substances Control Act.* GAO; 2013.

50. Jacobs J. *Eat to Heal.* Amazon Publishing; 2024.

51. Entani, E., Asai, M., Tsujihata, S., Tsukamoto, Y., & Ohta, M. (1998). Antibacterial action of vinegar against food borne pathogenic bacteria including *Escherichia coli* O157:H7. *Journal of Food Protection, 61*(8), 953–959. https://doi.org/10.4315/0362-028X-61.8.953

52. Farmer, V. C., Lumsdon, D. G., & Paterson, E. (2013). The role of sodium bicarbonate in surface cleaning and odor neutralization. *Journal of Environmental Health, 75*(6), 16–21.

References

53. Johnston, C. S., & Gaas, C. A. (2006). Vinegar: Medicinal uses and antimicrobial effects. *MedGenMed, 8*(2), 61.

54. Kampf, G. (2018). Efficacy of ethanol against viruses in hand disinfection. *Journal of Hospital Infection, 98*(4), 331–338. https://doi.org/10.1016/j.jhin.2017.08.025

55. McDonnell, G., & Russell, A. D. (1999). Antiseptics and disinfectants: Activity, action, and resistance. *Clinical Microbiology Reviews, 12*(1), 147–179.

56. Nazaroff, W. W., & Weschler, C. J. (2004). Cleaning products and air fresheners: Exposure to primary and secondary air pollutants. *Atmospheric Environment, 38*(18), 2841–2865.

57. Steinemann, A., Wargocki, P., & Rismanchi, B. (2017). Ten questions concerning fragrance free policies and indoor environments. *Building and Environment, 111*, 178–186.

58. U.S. Environmental Protection Agency. (2021). Safer choice standard and safer cleaning ingredients. https://www.epa.gov/saferchoice

59. Lessenger JE. Occupational acute anaphylactic reaction to assault by perfume spray in the face. *J Am Board Fam Pract.* 2001;14(2):137-140.

60. Senthilkumaran S, Meenakshisundaram R, Michaels AD, Balamurgan N, Thirumalaikolundusubramanian P. Ventricular fibrillation after exposure to air freshener: death just a breath away. *J Electrocardiol.* 2012;45(2):164-166. doi:10.1016/j.jelectrocard.2011.05.002

61. Hitosugi M, Tsukada C, Yamauchi S, et al. An autopsy case of fatal repellent air freshener poisoning. *Leg Med (Tokyo).* 2015;17(5):360-363. doi:10.1016/j.legalmed.2015.04.004

62. Centers for Disease Control and Prevention. CDC identifies rare bacteria in aromatherapy product. October 22, 2021.

63. U.S. Consumer Product Safety Commission. Walmart recalls Better Homes and Gardens essential oil infused aromatherapy room spray with gemstones due to rare and dangerous bacteria. November 2, 2021.

64. California Department of Public Health, Work-Related Asthma Prevention Program. *Fragrances and Work-Related Asthma: Information for Employers.* 2017.

65. Weinberg JL, Flattery J, Harrison R. Fragrances and work-related asthma: California surveillance data, 1993–2012. *J Asthma.* 2017;54(10):1041-1050. doi:10.1080/02770903.2017.1299755

66. Steinemann A. Fragranced consumer products: exposures and effects from emissions. *Air Qual Atmos Health.* 2016;9(8):861–866.

67. Steinemann A, MacGregor IC, Gordon SM, et al. Fragranced consumer products: chemicals emitted, ingredients unlisted. *Environ Impact Assess Rev.* 2011;31(3):328–333.

68. Doty RL. Olfactory system: overview. In: Doty RL, ed. *Handbook of Olfaction and Gustation.* 2nd ed. New York, NY: Marcel Dekker; 2001:3–28.

69. Herz RS. Aromatherapy facts and fictions: a scientific analysis of olfactory effects on mood, physiology and behavior. *Int J Neurosci.* 2009;119(2):263–290.

70. Woolf CJ. Central sensitization: implications for the diagnosis and treatment of pain. *Pain.* 2011;152(3 Suppl):S2–S15.

71. Caress SM, Steinemann AC. Prevalence of fragrance sensitivity in the American population. *J Environ Health.* 2009;71(7):46–50.

72. Anderson RC, Anderson JH. Acute toxicity of synthetic fragrances to aquatic organisms. *Arch Environ Contam Toxicol.* 1998;35(1):138–142.

73. Diamanti-Kandarakis E, Bourguignon JP, Giudice LC, et al. Endocrine-disrupting chemicals: an Endocrine Society scientific statement. *Endocr Rev.* 2009;30(4):293–342.

74. Landrigan PJ, Fuller R, Acosta NJR, et al. The Lancet Commission on pollution and health. *Lancet.* 2018;391(10119):462–512.

75. Miller CS, Prihoda TJ, Pollock B. Sensory hyperreactivity to volatile chemicals in multiple chemical sensitivity. *Toxicol Ind Health.* 2007;23(9):533–545.

References

76. Meggs WJ. Neurogenic inflammation and sensitivity to environmental chemicals. *Environ Health Perspect.* 1995;103(Suppl 6):234–238.
77. Purdue University. Air inside your home may be more polluted than outside due to everyday chemical products. 2025.
78. EWG. Valentine's Day: showing love for you or another with the perfect fragrance gift. 2026.
79. NIH. Certain chemicals may trigger early puberty in girls. 2024.
80. Burkart Y. Human study linking fragrance biomarkers to miscarriage. 2025.
81. FDA Unified Regulatory Agenda. Key updates for cosmetics. 2025.
82. IFRA. Fragrance allergen compliance 2026: IFRA 51/52, EU expansion. 2025.
83. Regulation (EU) 2023/1545. Amending cosmetic allergen labeling. 2023.
84. Steinemann A. Fragranced consumer products: exposures and effects from emissions. *Air Qual Atmos Health.* 2016;9(8):861–866. doi:10.1007/s11869-016-0442-z
85. Caress SM, Steinemann AC. Prevalence of fragrance sensitivity in the American population. *J Environ Health.* 2009;71(7):46–50.
86. Health Canada. Indoor Air Quality: Scent-Free Policies. Government of Canada; 2018.
87. Canadian Centre for Occupational Health and Safety. *Scent-Free Workplace Policies.* CCOHS; 2019.
88. Safe Work Australia. Workplace Air Quality and Chemical Exposure. Commonwealth of Australia; 2020.
89. Steinemann A. International prevalence of fragrance sensitivity. *Air Qual Atmos Health.* 2018;11(8):891–897. doi:10.1007/s11869-018-0607-9
90. NHS England. Creating a Scent-Free Healthcare Environment. National Health Service; 2019.
91. Azuma K, Uchiyama I, Tanigawa M, Bamba I. Chemical sensitivity and indoor air quality. *Int J Hyg Environ Health.* 2015;218(1):71–80. doi:10.1016/j.ijheh.2014.07.003
92. European Chemicals Agency. Guidance on Fragrance Allergens and Chemical Safety. ECHA; 2021.
93. U.S. Access Board. Indoor Environmental Quality and Accessibility. Access Board; 2020.
94. Diamanti-Kandarakis E, Bourguignon JP, Giudice LC, et al. Endocrine-disrupting chemicals: an endocrine society scientific statement. *Endocr Rev.* 2009;30(4):293–342.
95. International Agency for Research on Cancer. *Benzene.* IARC Monographs. 2018.
96. International Agency for Research on Cancer. *Formaldehyde.* IARC Monographs. 2012.
97. International Agency for Research on Cancer. *Titanium Dioxide.* IARC Monographs. 2010.
98. International Agency for Research on Cancer. *Carbon Black.* IARC Monographs. 2010.
99. International Agency for Research on Cancer. *Styrene.* IARC Monographs. 2019.
100. Smith MT. Advances in understanding benzene health effects and susceptibility. *Annu Rev Public Health.* 2010;31:133–148.
101. Steenland K, Whelan E, Deddens J, Stayner L, Ward E. Ethylene oxide and breast cancer incidence in a cohort study of 7576 women. *Cancer Causes Control.* 2004;15(5):531–539.
102. Americans with Disabilities Act of 1990, 42 U.S.C. § 12101 et seq.
103. Equal Employment Opportunity Commission. Enforcement guidance on reasonable accommodation and undue hardship under the ADA. Updated October 17, 2002.
104. Brady v. United Refrigeration, Inc., No. 13-6009, 2015 WL 3500125 (E.D. Pa. June 2, 2015).
105. Core v. Champaign County Board of County Commissioners, No. 3:11-cv-801, 2012 WL 3078814 (S.D. Ohio July 30, 2012).
106. McBride v. City of Detroit, No. 10-13506, 2011 WL 6118563 (E.D. Mich. Dec. 8, 2011).
107. Bester K. Analysis of musk fragrances in environmental samples. J Chromatogr A. 2009;1216(3):470-480.

References

108.European Chemicals Agency. Musk xylene and musk ketone risk assessment report. ECHA; 2010.

109.Luckenbach T, Epel D. Nitromusk and polycyclic musk compounds as long term inhibitors of cellular xenobiotic defense systems mediated by multidrug transporters. Environ Health Perspect. 2005;113(1):17-24.

110.Reiner JL, Kannan K. Polycyclic musks in human adipose tissue and breast milk. Environ Sci Technol. 2006;40(12):3813-3818.

111.Schreurs RHMM, Sonneveld E, Jansen JHJ, et al. Interaction of polycyclic musks with the estrogen receptor in vitro. Toxicol Sci. 2004;79(2):257-266.